COMPLETELY REVISED AND UPDATED

think
like a
pancreas

A PRACTICAL GUIDE TO
MANAGING DIABETES
WITH INSULIN

Gary Scheiner, MS, CDE

Foreword by Stanley Schwartz, MD

Da Capo
LIFE
LONG

A Member of the Perseus Books Group

Text design by Trish Wilkinson
Set in 11.5 point Goudy Old Style

Cataloging-in-Publication data for this book is available from the Library of Congress.

First Da Capo Press edition 2011
ISBN: 978-0-7382-1514-3

Published by Da Capo Press
A Member of the Perseus Books Group
www.dacapopress.com

Note: The information in this book is true and complete to the best of our knowledge. This book is intended only as an informative guide for those wishing to know more about health issues. In no way is this book intended to replace, countermand, or conflict with the advice given to you by your own physician. The ultimate decision concerning care should be made between you and your doctor. We strongly recommend you follow his or her advice. Information in this book is general and is offered with no guarantees on the part of the authors or Da Capo Press. The authors and publisher disclaim all liability in connection with the use of this book. The names and identifying details of people associated with events described in this book have been changed. Any similarity to actual persons is coincidental.

Da Capo Press books are available at special discounts for bulk purchases in the U.S. by corporations, institutions, and other organizations. For more information, please contact the Special Markets Department at the Perseus Books Group, 2300 Chestnut Street, Suite 200, Philadelphia, PA, 19103, or call (800) 810-4145, ext. 5000, or e-mail special.markets@perseusbooks.com.

10 9 8 7 6 5 4 3 2 1

What others are saying about
Think Like a Pancreas

"Gary Scheiner knows as much about diabetes as most endocrinologists and he has translated his knowledge and experience into a well-written, easy-to-read treatise on diabetes. A must-read for anyone with an interest in diabetes—most importantly patients and their families."
—STEVEN B. NAGELBERG, MD, CLINICAL ENDOCRINOLOGIST

"*Think Like a Pancreas* is delightful, unique, comprehensive, and detail oriented. The writing style is easy to follow. It will enlighten and educate for sure. Great work, Gary."
—PAULA HARPER, FOUNDER AND PRESIDENT
OF THE DIABETES EXERCISE AND SPORTS ASSOCIATION

"Gary Scheiner offers the missing 'manual' designed to benefit every patient with diabetes who wishes not only to optimize his/her self-care, but also to comprehend all the forces that work against easily achieving this lofty goal. He offers guidance, expertise, and a first-hand understanding of what it means to have to 'think like a pancreas.'"
—RENEE BERNETT, MOTHER OF A CHILD WITH TYPE I DIABETES
AND MEMBER OF THE JUVENILE DIABETES RESEARCH
FOUNDATION'S LAY REVIEW COMMITTEE

"*Think Like a Pancreas* is the most helpful guide that I've encountered about the intricacies of using insulin. Gary Scheiner speaks as one of us—someone who's lived with diabetes for nearly twenty years—and is able to translate sophisticated scientific concepts into clear laymen's terms. His humor is motivational and his understanding of the frustrations that can come with using insulin is truly encouraging. Though I've taken insulin on a daily basis for over twenty-three years, *Think Like a Pancreas* has opened my eyes to many new nuances that will surely help me—and countless other people with diabetes—in my quest for tight blood sugar control."
—GABRIELLE KAPLAN-MAYER, AUTHOR OF
Insulin Pump Therapy Demystified, WWW.INSULINPUMPBOOK.COM

To MJ, Bumble Bee, Awesome Boy,
Lily Poppins, and The Princess.
And to my wife, Debbie,
who let me live long enough to finish this book.

Contents

CHAPTER 9

Going to Extremes   219

CHAPTER 10

Resources for Everything and Anything Diabetes   251

Foreword

No man is an island, entire of itself; every man is a piece of the continent.

— JOHN DONNE

The nice thing about teamwork is that you always have others on your side.

— MARGARET CARTY

Achieving excellent control of diabetes is a difficult task for any individual. This is because so many factors influence blood glucose levels as well as the potential for adverse outcomes. Diabetes affects many different parts of the body, and there are biologic differences within each individual. Add to that the fact that each person reacts differently to insulin, medication, diet, exercise, emotional states, and physical stresses. Nevertheless, there is no doubt that excellent diabetes control reduces eye, kidney, and nerve disease as well as heart attacks, strokes, and amputations, all while improving the quality of one's daily life.

It is impossible for any singular physician to "know" everything about diabetes—one needs metabolism and general medical expertise as well as often, sadly, ophthalmology, cardiovascular, kidney, podiatry, and neurology expertise. Although the endocrinologist with experience in diabetes can be a conductor among the physicians, he frequently needs help.

Similarly, the individual living with diabetes can't easily become an expert in nutrition, exercise, stress, technology, and the myriad other topics involved in diabetes self-care. Everyone must recognize that they need some help. Each patient needs nurses, nutritionists, exercise physiologists, mental health counselors, and Certified Diabetes Educators to help achieve the goal of excellent glucose control. Thus, *teamwork* is key.

One of most difficult aspects of controlling glucose is the self-adjustment of insulin. One must adapt insulin doses to all aspects of daily life—diet, exercise, stress, and so on. With this in mind, Gary Scheiner has written this book. It is for all team members—from the patient to the diabetes educator to the primary care and specialized physician—who need to master basic principles and advanced techniques in the use of insulin.

Mr. Scheiner has updated his successful first edition, continuing to emphasize the establishment of an appropriate basal/bolus insulin program and the fine tuning of said doses. This edition also focuses on several new approaches, including the use of continuous glucose monitoring, glucose management during pregnancy, use of newer medications, and all of the latest diabetes self-care technologies.

He is eminently qualified to do so given his experience with patients of all ages—children, teens, and adults; his training as an exercise physiologist; his publications on pump therapy, continuous glucose monitoring, women's issues (control during the menstrual cycle and pregnancy), behavioral issues, and nutrition; his awards from the ADA and AADE recognizing his teaching expertise; and his lectures to audiences nationally and internationally. Moreover, as a type 1 patient himself for more than twenty-five years, he has the unique opportunity to translate his personal experience to those fortunate enough to be clients of his practice, members of his audiences, and readers of this book.

We as physicians who care for these patients are privileged to have Gary write a book such as this and to have him on our team. He is the ultimate team player. And when we work as a team, everyone wins.

Stanley Schwartz, MD
Affiliate, Main Line Health System
Clinical Associate Professor, Emeritus
University of Pennsylvania,
Ardmore, Pennsylvania
June 2011

1

Let's Get Acquainted

Let's be upfront. Either you forked down good money for this book or somebody is making you read it. Either way, you've invested your time and/or money and deserve to get something good in return.

So how do you know you can trust little, old me to set you on the golden path to better diabetes management? I find that establishing some common ground helps. For starters, I too find diabetes to be a royal pain in the butt (pain in the bum for those of you in EU and AU; pain in the tuchus for my Israeli friends). The whole idea of working at something year after year only so that nothing *bad* happens just doesn't sit well with me. And even after working at it, the results aren't always there. Why, for instance, can the same type of bagel from the same shop make my glucose go very high one day but not the next?

Like you, I have enough to do without all the added responsibilities of taking care of my diabetes. Doctor's visits, getting lab work, and treating lows take time away that I'd much rather spend with my wife or kids. Checking blood glucose, counting carbs, and calculating insulin doses are part of the price we all have to pay before eating just about anything. And speaking of price, I'd much rather spend my money on new clothes or tickets to a ballgame than on CGM sensors and pump supplies. Heck, managing diabetes is like having another entire job lopped on top of everything else in our lives—but without weekends off, and certainly without the moolah.

You may have also found, as I have, that today's health care system simply isn't equipped to manage diabetes properly. And that goes for more than just the American system; virtually everyone I've consulted across the globe has had the same experience: Health care providers consistently come up short when it comes to time, expertise, and access. This is not from a lack of desire; most physicians are talented, motivated, caring people who wish they had the time and resources to do more for their patients. It's just that the demands placed on today's physicians (and their support staff) are so great that precious little time is available for teaching/helping us learn the finer points of living with diabetes. And this is true whether your clinician is part of a government-funded health program, a managed-care organization, or a private group of health care providers.

Hopefully, you're nodding your head by now, mumbling "Yea, he *gets* it." Well, here's a synopsis of my life with diabetes thus far. See if anything else sounds familiar.

My Story

It was two o'clock in the afternoon on a typically hot, muggy summer day in Sugarland, Texas, a suburb in southwest Houston. (No, I'm not making this up. The irony is just unbelievable.) After spending half the summer sucking down cold drinks and the other half peeing them out, I decided it was time to see the family doctor.

I hardly knew this doctor, but I had had about all I could take. My energy was gone, and there was no way the Houston summer could have caused me to lose so much weight—I had gone from 155 pounds to 117. I actually couldn't tighten my belt enough to keep my pants from falling down. Then I saw an episode of M*A*S*H in which a helicopter pilot had diabetes. And guess what: He had many of the same symptoms! So I decided it was time to get checked out.

The doctor's office was only a ten-minute drive from my family's house, so I was able to make it with just one pit stop to use a gas sta-

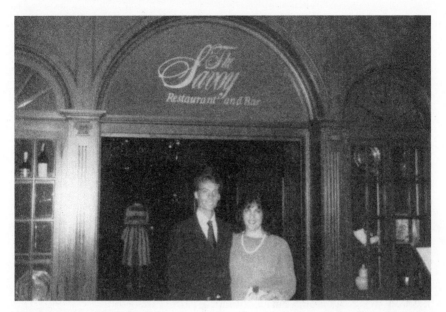

The clothes hanger on the left is me, out on a formal date the night of my diagnosis, forty pounds underweight.

tion restroom. (That summer, I learned where all the best public rest-rooms were along the I-59 corridor in southwest Houston.) When I got to the doctor's office, I put on my glasses (miraculously, I could sud-denly see road signs *without* my glasses for the first time ever), wiped off the steam created by the 10,000 percent humidity, and prepared myself for the worst.

After a quick physical exam, blood test, and urinalysis, the doctor came back in and said nonchalantly, "Gary, I've got good news and I've got bad news. The bad news is that you have diabetes, and you're going to have it for the rest of your life."

I have no idea what the good news was because I stopped listening at that point. The first syllable from "diabetes" stuck in my head. What the heck is *diabetes*? About all I knew was that it was making my body wither away and that it wasn't going to go away until I died.

I remember him telling me that my blood sugar was 600-something, and that that was six times the normal level. I also remember him saying that I would have to take shots and be very careful about what I ate. The thought of giving myself shots was one thing, but limit what I eat? Was he crazy? I was an active eighteen-year-old with the metabolism of a small country. The very thought of not being able to eat whatever I wanted whenever I wanted made me more depressed than anything else.

So off I went to an endocrinologist at a fancy high-rise in downtown Houston. Keep in mind that the year was 1985 and there were no HMOs yet, so getting in to see a specialist was as easy as making a phone call.

"You are lucky to be diagnosed now," explained the endocrinologist. "We have come a long way in the treatment of diabetes. I'll bet that in five or ten years, your diabetes will be cured."

I should have taken that bet.

I then met with a nurse who taught me the basics about diabetes. I discovered what insulin is and why it is important. I learned a little bit about how food and exercise affect blood sugar levels and what can happen if I don't keep mine under control. I also found out why the high blood sugars I had been experiencing all summer turned me into a human water fountain.

Finally, I was instructed on how to inject insulin. Forget about practicing on oranges, pillows, and teddy bears. I gave myself my very first injection, right in the stomach. It hurt, probably because I had almost no fat left on my body and the syringe needles were much thicker and longer than they are today. But mostly it hurt because I was tense and overwhelmed at the thought of sticking needles in myself for the rest of my life.

I was also given a bottle of test strips and taught about blood sugar testing. No meter, mind you—just test strips. These strips had a big square box at the tip that had to be covered with blood, blotted, and then timed before matching the color on the strip to the color chart on the bottle. Pale blue meant you were 40 to 70 mg/dl (a bit low); light blue, 70 to 100 (low to normal); ocean blue, 100 to 125 (normal); aqua-blue, 125 to 150 (slightly above normal); just plain aqua, 150 to 200 (a bit too high); aqua-green, 200 to 250 (high); sea green, 250 to 350 (very high); green, 350 to 450 (very, very high); brownish green, look out. In other words, determining your blood sugar required an extremely sensitive eye for subtle differences in pastels. Hey . . . when I grew up, there were only eight crayons in my box of Crayolas, and none of them were "sea green."

The bottle of test strips came with a medieval torture device called an "Autolet." The Autolet had a small disposable platform with a hole where you placed the victim . . . er . . . I mean, your finger. A disposable twenty-five-gauge lancet was placed in the firing mechanism, which swung around at a high speed like a pendulum to stab your finger and make it bleed. I called it "The Guillotine."

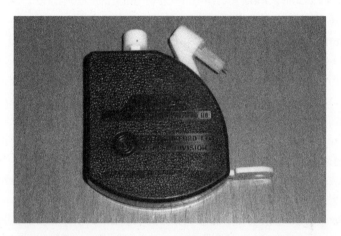

The original "guillotine" (I mean Autolet) for performing fingersticks.

Then I met with a dietitian—a tiny, middle-aged woman who taught me the fine art of the "exchange" diet.

"You really don't have to change what you eat that much," she told me. "You just have to be careful not to eat too many concentrated sweets, fats, or very large portions of anything." Apparently, she had no idea who she was talking to.

I can still remember my "generous" 2,500-calorie exchange diet—chock-full of fruits, vegetables, meats, milks, fats, and starches. Oh, how I hated that diet sheet. I was hungry constantly. The exchange system meant that everything I ate had to be placed in a category and that I could only eat so many things from each category at each meal and snack. Talk about sucking all the fun out of eating!

My first "exchange diet" meal looked so puny on the plate—a sandwich, a piece of fruit, a cup of milk, and a handful of chips. And there were no seconds, thirds, or fourths like I was used to having. I was hungry *all* the time.

The first couple of weeks were really rough. Even after starving myself and doing everything I was asked to do, the stupid test strips kept turning aqua-blue instead of sea green (or maybe it was the other way around). I cried a lot those first couple of weeks. My mom told me that my dad, normally an unemotional guy (a chemical engineer by trade), was crying too, and that he wished it was him and not me who got diabetes.

A few weeks after my diagnosis I purchased my first blood glucose meter—a Glucometer, to be exact. It weighed about a pound and was the size of a sandwich, but without the onion smell. The testing procedure is still etched in my brain: Guillotine, then squeeze out a big "hanging" drop of blood, dab the big box on the strip, start the counter, wait one minute, blot the strip and insert it in the meter, press the button again, and wait ninety seconds for that 58 or 314 to appear. (Just once, wouldn't you like to see a meter advertisement in which the reading on the screen wasn't so darned *perfect*?)

That meter lasted about a year. Then Lifescan came out with its first One Touch meter, and I jumped to get one. Imagine—no blotting, a round test area (covering a square box with a round drop is not

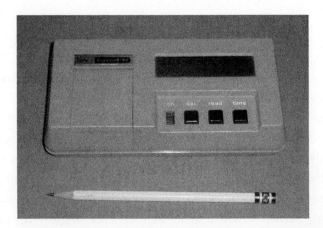

My first blood glucose meter, aka "the brick."

easy!), and only forty-five seconds from stick to finish. I was in hyperglycemic heaven. It didn't do much for my control, but I did have an extra five minutes a day to spend doing things other than waiting for my test results.

My early insulin program presented another challenge: NPH and regular, at breakfast and dinner. NPH was the long-acting insulin in vogue at that time; regular was the stuff used to cover meals. The regular would peak in about two hours and last about six; the NPH would peak in six hours and last about twelve. Everyone at the endocrinologist's office kept telling me the same thing: "You can live a normal life as long as you do things according to your insulin." Basically, that meant that I would have to eat certain things at certain times of day, exercise (with caution) at certain times of day, sleep only at certain times because of the need to take shots at specific times, and test my blood sugar at certain times. What could be more normal than that?

Back in 1985, two shots a day was the norm. So was making your life conform to your insulin program. But things did improve over time. I was given a sliding scale for my insulin, which was a good thing because I began sneaking in lots of extra exchanges in my meals and snacks, and was rarely "ocean blue." With all the exercise I did, I probably had as many lows as I had highs, so my glycosylated hemoglobin levels showed a decent overall average, but the low blood sugars were becoming more frequent and more severe, especially during the night.

When I returned to college in the fall, my doctor suggested that I move my dinnertime NPH to bedtime. Although that helped cut down on the nighttime lows, I started having more lows before lunch. Oy vey.

My One Touch meter got a lot of use through college (I went to Washington University in Saint Louis, home of the Cardinals and the world's best frozen custard). Before dinner my friends in the dorm would gather to wager on my blood sugar level. Everyone threw a dollar on the table, with the closest guess taking the loot. Some of them became pretty adept at the whole diabetes thing: They would ask questions like, "What did you eat for lunch?" and "Did you work out this afternoon?" Talk about getting by with a little help from my friends! Lighthearted stuff like that kept me from getting down about my diabetes.

Despite the technological improvements, frequent high and low readings still plagued me. Anyone with diabetes knows how those blood sugar swings make you feel fatigued and frustrated. Besides the support of my friends, exercise was a key to helping me keep a positive attitude. I had always been into sports, but after being diagnosed with diabetes my passion for staying in shape soared to a whole new level. Every day I managed to find time for some form of exercise. If no one was available to play basketball or racquetball, I would go to the gym to work out, ride my bike around the park, or jump rope in the lounge to the beat of Motown music. Exercising made me feel like I was still strong, fit, and in control of my own health, despite having diabetes.

Unfortunately, a serious low blood sugar often followed the emotional high I got from exercise. One month after starting my first postcollege job, I showed up for work in a complete daze. Some days I couldn't even remember getting dressed or driving to work. That I never crashed buck-naked into a tree is amazing. To make matters worse, I was no longer getting symptoms that a low blood sugar was coming. Gone were the good old days of shakes and cold sweats. Now, mental confusion was the first noticeable sign that my blood sugar was dropping, and sometimes it was too late for me to handle it on my own.

Thank God for my wife, Debbie, who I met in college. She's very good at knowing when to let me do my own thing and when to get involved, and I knew I would marry her after our first Valentine's Day together. She learned a few things about diabetes and went out of her way to prepare a huge heart-shaped box filled with popcorn and pistachios. You know what they say . . . the way to a man's heart is through his pancreas.

Debbie and I left Saint Louis and moved to Chicago after we both graduated. While in Chicago I met with a few more endocrinologists and other specialists about my diabetes. By that time I was growing more and more frustrated with the constant swings between highs and lows. Nobody had any answers—just the same old rhetoric about "This is what your insulin is doing. You just need to adjust to it."

Then I had the most severe low blood sugar of my life. It came in the middle of the night after I had been playing full-court basketball earlier in the evening. According to Debbie, I was pale and completely un-responsive. My limbs jerked uncontrollably. She called for paramedics, and according to the reports, I fought them off pretty well while they tried to put an IV into my arm. When I finally regained consciousness, Debbie was standing next to me with an exhausted, worried look on her face. I looked to the side and saw tubes coming out of my arm. I also saw blood. My blood—on the pillow, on the sheets, on the floor—everywhere.

That experience really shook me up. Then I met an exercise physi-ologist who worked part time at a nearby diabetes clinic. He had dia-betes himself and gave me some suggestions about eating extra food at bedtime and self-adjusting my long-acting insulin to prevent the night-time lows after exercise. This was the first time anyone had introduced the concept of self-adjusting my insulin doses. Why hadn't my doctor told me about this?

That exercise physiologist opened my eyes to more than just how to adjust insulin by a few units (his recommendations worked very nicely, by the way); he set me on an entirely new career path. I liked his approach so much that I decided to become an exercise physiolo-gist for people with diabetes. So what if there were no full-time jobs for exercise physiologists at diabetes centers? I loved to exercise, I had diabetes, and I was on a mission to put the two together to help as many people as possible. So I went back to school, earned my master's degree in exercise physiology, and landed a position with the Joslin Diabetes Center's affiliate in Philadelphia.

Being a New York/New Jersey native, Philadelphia seemed close enough to home—and it had its own NBA, NFL, and Major League Baseball franchises (I don't think I could live in a city that did not have them). So we packed up and moved to Philly, where I became the Joslin Center's full-time exercise guru. I have to admit, my office was really cool. It had weights, treadmills, bikes, video equipment, and a great view of the sports complex in south Philly. The only thing better than my office was the clinical team with whom I worked. The doctors, nurses, dietitians, and psychologists were heavily into the concept of flexible insulin dosing and self-adjustment. I cross-trained with them at every opportunity and absorbed as much as I could about the many facets and nuances of diabetes care.

Perhaps the greatest breakthrough in my own self-care was my decision in 1994 to try an insulin pump. Nobody at our diabetes center had used one, but our patients expressed a mounting interest to have an insulin pump program. So I decided to be the guinea pig.

I'll never forget how nervous I was the day I got hooked up to that little gray box. There were about twenty doctors, nurses, and administrators watching my every move. My first infusion set was a steel needle (the needle actually stayed in all the time). Soon, a flexible plastic infusion set became available, followed by a set that could be disconnected and reconnected easily. Before that, you had to stay connected to the pump all the time—during showers, sports, even sex.

The pump was very basic compared to today's models. Nevertheless, simply having the ability to adjust basal insulin levels and mealtime boluses really helped to stabilize my blood sugar levels. For the first time in almost ten years I could sleep past 8 a.m. without having my blood sugar skyrocket. I could delay my lunch without bottoming out. And best of all was that I could work out to my heart's content without going low in the middle of the night. In fact, I haven't had a single severe low blood sugar since I started on the pump more than fifteen years ago.

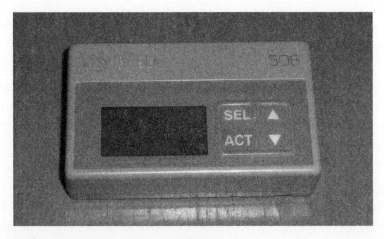

My first insulin pump, the MiniMed 506.

With pump therapy came a whole new approach to dietary management: carb counting. By counting the grams of carbohydrate in my meals and snacks, I can now eat what I choose as long as I match it with the correct dose of rapid-acting insulin. "Grazing" is still a problem; blood sugars tend to stay elevated if meals and snacks are consumed too often. So I try to spread my feedings several hours apart.

The introduction of rapid-acting insulin analogs (lispro, then aspart, then glulisine) starting in the late 1990s has had a tremendous impact on my diabetes management. Unlike regular insulin, which takes thirty minutes to start working, two to three hours to peak, and five to six hours to fade, the rapid-acting analogs peak in about an hour and only last three to four hours. They do the job and then get out of the way. A few years ago I added another injectable medication to my treatment program: pramlintide (Symlin). This hormone, produced by the beta cells of the pancreas (and lacking in those of us with type 1 diabetes) helps to slow down digestion so that blood sugars don't spike right after eating. The combination of rapid-acting insulin and Symlin has worked wonders. Gone are my 300-plus blood sugars right after eating; instead, the readings stay remarkably level between meals. I can also afford to be more spontaneous and flexible in terms of what and when I eat.

Of course, there have been a few other developments along the way. My blood glucose meter now takes less than one microliter of blood and performs the test in five seconds. An adjustable lancing pen with lancets that are micro-thin has replaced the old Guillotine. Using a sound lancing technique, I can barely feel the finger pricks anymore. If I choose, I can even take a reading from my arm or leg. I can do a Hemoglobin A1c in ten minutes with a machine that I have in my office, and virtually everything is downloadable. My latest insulin pump has so many advanced features that it can practically do my taxes for me!

And then there's my latest toy: the continuous glucose monitor (CGM). I began using CGM back in 2004, when the system was connected to your body by way of a cable and the information was kept secret until you took the sensor out of your body and downloaded the receiver to a computer. Since then, the accuracy has improved: They have gone wireless, they produce on-screen graphs and data for real-time use, and they sport a variety of customizable alerts to guard against high and low glucose levels.

Personally, I've found CGM to be the best thing since sliced sourdough bread (you'll learn about the magical powers of sourdough bread later on in this book). I love the fact that I don't have to prick my finger quite so often, and the alerts have saved me from many highs and lows. Perhaps the best thing about them is that they provide *context* to glucose values. Knowing you're 100 (5.5 mmol/l) is one thing; knowing that you're 100 and dropping or rising quickly is another. I was officially sold on CGM when I completed my first ten-mile run (the Broad Street Run in Philadelphia). I ran the entire course with my CGM receiver in my fist, checking as I approached each rest stop to see if I needed to grab water or Gatorade. My control was immaculate, and I finished the race without having to stop once.

But technology aside, the thing that has made the greatest difference in my life with diabetes is learning how to match my insulin to my needs. No more molding my life to fit my insulin program. Now I shape the insulin to fit the life I want to live. And that's what I try to teach my clients to do—to think like a pancreas!

As proud as I am of what we have accomplished in diabetes care and treatment, I can't help but recall how proud my original endocrinologist was with the state of things back in 1985. Twenty-five years from now, I'll probably look back to today and think, "Did we really do all *that* just to manage diabetes? That was totally archaic!"

At least I hope so.

Chapter Highlights _____

- I, like you, think diabetes is a royal pain.
- My diagnosis took place in 1985 in *Sugarland*, Texas. God's honest truth.
- Diabetes self-management has evolved considerably over the past several decades.

2

What's the Dang Diddly Point?*

Picture this: You show up for your regular appointment at the doctor's office. After the usual checkup, you report to the front desk, checkbook in hand, ready to pay for your visit. "Hold on," says the receptionist with a cheerful smile. "That won't be necessary. Here you go." She hands you an envelope stuffed with cash. "This is for all the work you've put in to taking care of your diabetes."

That's when the alarm clock goes off. Dream over.

> Taking care of diabetes is really just an ongoing series of small sacrifices, costs, mental efforts, and time commitments.

Taking care of yourself when you have diabetes takes serious work, and at times it may seem quite thankless. It's not punch-clock kind of work; rather, it's more of an ongoing series of small sacrifices, costs, mental efforts, and time commitments, with the occasional minor discomfort. So why do it? Even though you're not likely to get paid for

---

* paraphrasing Ned Flanders from *The Simpsons*

the work you put in, there are many valuable benefits you are likely to experience.

What's in It for Me Now?

We'll get to the long-term benefits of proper diabetes care a bit later on. What motivates most people is *immediate gratification*. Not tomorrow, not next year—*right now*. Here is just a partial list of ways you will be rewarded immediately for managing your diabetes. (I think you'll find it well worth the effort!)

Immediate Benefits of Diabetes Control

- increased energy
- more restful sleep
- improved physical performance
- appetite reduction
- brain power
- stable moods/emotions
- fewer sick days
- healthier skin and gums
- personal safety
- predictable menstrual cycles

Increased Energy

Raise your hand if you like being tired all the time. Okay, raise your hand if you're too tired to raise your hand. Elevated blood glucose reduces energy levels. High glucose is a sign that you may not be getting enough fuel into your body's cells to burn for energy. The fuel is there . . . it's just stuck in the bloodstream, kind of like gasoline trucks that drive around aimlessly instead of unloading at local gas stations. This shortage of fuel inside the body's cells causes sleepiness and sluggishness. Even if the glucose is only elevated temporarily, the lack of energy will be noticeable during that time. As soon as the level returns to normal, energy levels usually improve.

More Restful Sleep

We all know how important a good night's sleep is for feeling good and being productive the next day. Getting sufficient sleep is also linked to appetite control. Our production of the hunger-controlling hormone leptin is diminished when sleep is inadequate.

It may interest you to know that poor glucose control reduces the *quality* of sleep. If your glucose is high enough (typically above 180 mg/dl, or 10 mmol/l), you might wake up several times during the night to run to the bathroom. This is caused by *urine diuresis*. When glucose levels are elevated, the kidneys have a hard time keeping all that extra sugar in the bloodstream. Sugar spills over into the urine, and it drags a lot of water along with it. As the bladder fills, it wakes us up and leads to those middle-of-the-night two-minute, sugar-induced peeing sessions. If the thought of a restful, uninterrupted night's sleep appeals to you, control your diabetes!

Improved Physical Performance

Whether you're an aspiring athlete or just hoping to make it up a flight of stairs without losing your lunch, glucose control has an immediate effect on your physical abilities. Elevated glucose can reduce your strength, flexibility, speed, stamina, and endurance.

> Keeping blood sugar near normal will result in improved strength, speed, flexibility, and endurance.

Sugar is our muscles' favorite fuel for making short, rapid movements, so limiting access to sugar is a detriment to one's strength. Extra sugar in the bloodstream also leads to something called *glycosylation*—sticking of sugar to connective tissues like tendons and ligaments, thus limiting their ability to stretch properly. Muscle stiffness, strains, and pulls are common in people with high blood sugar levels. High sugars block the connection between muscles and nerves, resulting in slower reaction times and reflexes. Extra sugar in the bloodstream limits our red blood cells' ability to pick up oxygen in the lungs and transport it to our muscles. This can cause fatigue and limited cardiovascular/aerobic capacity. Dehydration and cramping are also common side effects of hyperglycemia (high blood sugar).

When glucose levels are near normal, your reaction times will be quicker and you will recover from injuries more rapidly. Many of my clients have tracked their performance in a variety of sports and have consistently performed best when their blood glucose is in the 80–140 mg/dl range (4.5–8 mmol/l). One young man's first MVP trophy in an ice hockey tournament coincided with the first time he managed to keep his blood sugar from going high or low throughout (we'll discuss details regarding sports/exercise control later on). Overall, you're likely to see improved performance in all sorts of activities—from carrying groceries to playing soccer to lovemaking—when your blood sugars remain near normal.

Appetite Reduction

This might sound totally bass-ackwards, but high glucose levels tend to make us crave more food, especially carbohydrate-rich foods. Remember, the amount of sugar in the bloodstream is not what counts but rather how much gets into our cells, and if not enough is getting into our cells, our hunger will increase. So controlling glucose levels is a good way to keep your appetite in check.

Brain Power

High and low glucose limits our ability to focus, remember, perform complex tasks, and be creative. Research studies have repeatedly and consistently shown that as blood sugars go up, so do mental errors and the time it takes to perform basic tasks. Wide variations in blood sugar levels, such as postmeal spikes, have also been shown to hinder intellectual function. Likewise, if glucose levels are too low (typically below 55 mg/dl, or 3 mmol/l), the entire nervous system lacks the fuel it needs to operate correctly. So if you want to perform as well as possible at work, in school, or in a friendly game of Guitar Hero, watch those sugar levels.

Stable Moods and Emotions

Besides intellectual performance, the brain is also responsible for maintaining our emotional balance. The fact is our moods often change along with our blood sugars. If you don't believe me, ask those around you! (My wife didn't take long to realize that.) High glucose levels can make us impatient, irritable, and generally negative. Achieving normal blood sugars *and keeping them there* can go a long way toward improving your mood and emotional stability. This is not to say that you will become an instant socialite, but the way you interact with your family, friends, coworkers, classmates, and even perfect strangers can impact your happiness and success in life.

Fewer Sick Days

Bacteria and viruses *love* sugar. They gobble it up and use it to grow and multiply. When blood glucose levels are up, the amount of sugar in virtually all of our body's tissues and fluids rises as well. This makes us ideal breeding grounds for infection. Think of it as "aiding and abetting the enemy"—supplying extra nutrients to the bad guys. Everything from common colds to sinus infections to flu and vaginal yeast infections are more common when blood sugars are elevated. And once illnesses and infections set in, they are much harder to shake when the blood sugar is high. Research has shown that people with better blood sugar control spend significantly fewer days absent from work, sick in bed, and restricted from their usual activities. So if you want to keep from getting sick, take better care of your diabetes!

Softer Skin, Healthier Gums

Two body parts that changes in glucose levels affect immediately are the skin and gums. Our level of hydration greatly influences our skin. When blood sugars are high, skin tends to become dry and cracked. This can not only be uncomfortable and unsightly, but it also sets us up for potential infections because the skin is the first line of defense against harmful bacteria. Keeping glucose levels in control helps to prevent dehydration and keep our skin soft and intact.

Changes in sugar levels also immediately affect our gums. Bacteria that live below the gum line grow quickly when exposed to high sugar levels in our blood vessels. These bacteria then form plaque at an accelerated rate, contributing to bleeding gums and loose teeth. Controlling your diabetes will help cut back on plaque buildup immediately.

Personal Safety

If you happen to drive a car, operate power equipment, play a sport, or just walk across the street from time to time, having out-of-control blood sugar can put you and those around you at risk. We have already discussed how high glucose can cause sleepiness and slow reaction times (a recipe for disaster when driving), but the opposite extreme—*hypoglycemia* (low blood sugar)—can be even more dangerous. Hypoglycemia can occur in anyone taking insulin, even if it's just once daily. Below-normal glucose levels will usually cause a surge of adrenaline and some degree of temporary brain impairment. Decision making and judgment will be off. Coordination suffers, and trembling can occur. To keep yourself and those around you safe, you must manage your blood sugar properly.

Predictable Menstrual Cycles

Research has shown that women with near-normal HbA1c levels tend to have more consistent, regular menstrual cycles than do women with an elevated A1c. And with predictability comes power. As you will learn later in this book, the ability to predict events that influence glucose levels allows us the opportunity to make effective adjustments.

What's in It for Me Later?

We all know of someone who has (or had) diabetes and wound up going blind, losing a foot, or needing to go on dialysis for failing kidneys. If not, someone is sure to come along and ever-so-delicately share a diabetes horror story with you. If the thought of your vital organs decaying and body parts falling off bothers you, then *good*: Fear and anger can be powerful motivators. They are what keep us from doing stupid things like picking fights with people twice our size, and they give us the power to take on someone who might be trying to hurt us or our kids. Use it as your "management fuel."

> Let the fear and anger associated with long-term diabetic complications serve as a positive motivator.

Long-Term Benefits of Blood Sugar Control

- healthy eyes
- healthy kidneys
- a strong heart
- adequate blood flow
- proper nerve function
- protective nerve sensation
- minimal pain
- healthy feet
- intact memory
- flexible joints
- mental health
- successful pregnancy

One might think that sugar is a good thing—it sure tastes good! But too much of a good thing is, well, not so good. Glucose levels that are too high over a period of many years cause damage to virtually every major system of the body. But there is good news. Major long-term multicenter research projects such as the Diabetes Control and Complications Trial (DCCT) and the United Kingdom Prospective Diabetes Study (UKPDS) have proven beyond a reasonable doubt that *tight glucose control does make a difference.*

Maintaining a hemoglobin A1c (HbA1c, or simply A1c) as close to normal as possible has been shown to greatly reduce the health risks associated with diabetes over the long term. Likewise, minimizing glucose variability (dramatic swings into high and low glucose ranges) is believed to have a stabilizing effect on blood vessels and the organs they nourish.

Of course, there are going to be some ups and downs when it comes to your blood sugar levels; we're not yet at the point at which *perfection* is possible. But over the long term, if you take good care of your diabetes, here's what you can most likely look forward to:

Keen Eyesight

In the back of the eye is a sensitive layer called the retina. Like the film in a camera, the retina receives light from the outside world and transmits signals to the brain to produce vision. Many small blood vessels (capillaries) provide the living cells of the retina with oxygen and nutrients, but elevated blood sugar levels make these capillaries very fragile. The capillaries can swell, leak, or grow in unhealthy ways, thereby blocking light from reaching the retina. This is called *diabetic retinopathy*.

Diabetes is the leading cause of blindness among adults aged twenty to seventy-four. Diabetic retinopathy accounts for approximately twenty thousand cases of blindness each year. Glaucoma, cataracts, and corneal disease are also more common in people with diabetes, and they contribute to the high rate of blindness.

The good news is that tight blood sugar control reduces the risk of retinopathy. The DCCT trial showed a 30 percent reduction in the risk of developing retinopathy for every one-point reduction in A1c, corresponding with approximately a 30 mg/dl or 1.7 mmol/l reduction in average blood glucose. And for those with existing retinopathy, tightening blood sugar control slows the progression significantly.

Fabulous Filters

Visit any kidney dialysis center and check the charts of the people who sit there for hours every week with tubes in their arms so that their blood can be siphoned out, pumped through machines, and filtered clean. You'll see: diabetic, diabetic, not diabetic, diabetic, diabetic.

You get the idea.

Diabetes is the leading cause of kidney failure. Approximately fifty thousand Americans with diabetes begin treatment for end-stage renal disease each year. Elevated blood sugar does damage to the tiny blood vessels (capillaries) that form and nourish the filters within the kidneys. *The good news* is that tightening blood sugar control reduces the risk of kidney disease dramatically. As was the case with retinopathy, every 30 mg/dl (1.7) drop in average blood sugar leads to a 30 percent reduction in kidney disease risk.

Heart Health

Despite the long list of health problems diabetes can cause, heart disease is what ultimately kills the majority of people with diabetes. People with diabetes are two to four times more likely to develop heart disease and five times more likely to *die* from heart disease compared to people without diabetes. Why? Having excessive amounts of sugar in the bloodstream causes problems. Sugar is a sticky substance (think of the last time you ate cotton candy or spilled some juice). It makes things like cholesterol stick to the walls of blood vessels, thereby causing the formation of plaques. These plaques make the blood vessels thick and rigid, a condition known as *atherosclerosis*. When pieces of the plaques break off, clots can develop, and these restrict blood flow to vital organs such as the heart.

The good news is that improving blood sugar control reduces the risk of heart disease dramatically. Besides eliminating a great deal of the cement that clogs up blood vessels, it can also lead to reductions in cholesterol and blood pressure levels. And don't forget: The things we do to control blood sugar, such as exercising, eating healthier, and cutting back on stress, also reduce our risk for heart disease.

Sound Circulation

Besides the heart, a number of other body parts require large amounts of oxygen and nutrients. The brain, for example: When blood vessels leading to the brain become clogged, the brain does not receive enough oxygen, and then brain cells begin to die. This is called a *stroke*. The risk of stroke is two to four times higher among people with diabetes.

The muscles in the legs also depend on significant blood flow, particularly during exercise. When blood vessels serving the leg muscles become clogged and oxygen delivery is limited, pain or cramping can occur when exercising, walking, or simply standing. This condition is called *claudication*. Blood vessel disease in the legs is *twenty times* more common in people with diabetes, and some degree of claudication occurs in 45 percent of people who have had diabetes for more than twenty years.

Again, *the good news* is that tightening blood sugar control, along with all the other lifestyle improvements that come with it, will improve circulation to vital body parts.

All Systems Go

Our nervous system, for lack of a better phrase, serves as the wiring for our bodies. More specifically, the autonomic portion of our nervous system controls the behind-the-scenes functions that are going on—things like heart rate, digestion, temperature regulation, balance, and sexual function.

Nerves are like any other living tissue in the body: They burn sugar for energy and require a blood supply for oxygen and nutrients. Elevated blood sugar levels seem to cause two problems for nerves: They interfere with the blood supply, and energy metabolism is altered such that the nerves swell and lose the waxy coating that normally provides insulation for the nerve fibers. Damage to the nerves that regulate basic body functions is called *autonomic neuropathy*.

Population-based studies have shown that 60 to 70 percent of people with diabetes will develop some form of nerve damage in their lifetime. Nearly 50 percent of all men with diabetes develop impotency, due mainly to malfunction of the nerves that produce an erection. Women with diabetes are more likely than nondiabetic women to suffer from vaginal dryness. Delayed digestion (gastroparesis) affects nearly 30 percent of people with diabetes. This condition can cause painful bloating, and the extremely slow rate of digestion can make diabetes even more difficult to control. Postural hypotension (low blood pressure upon sitting or standing) is twice as common in people with diabetes.

The good news is that blood sugar control is an effective means for preventing all forms of autonomic neuropathy. And here's more good news for those who already have neuropathy: Although it is not always reversible, the condition may regress slightly or cease to progress further once blood sugar levels return toward normal.

Freedom from Pain

As mentioned above, 60 to 70 percent of all people with diabetes develop some form of nerve damage in their lifetime. Most develop a form called *peripheral neuropathy*—malfunction of the nerves leading to the extremities such as the feet and lower legs. In its early stages peripheral neuropathy takes the form of tingling or numbness. But as it progresses and nerve inflammation develops, it can cause constant and sometimes severe pain. Although there are many medical and alternative medicine treatments for painful neuropathy, many people find little or no relief.

The good news is that tight blood sugar control can help to minimize the pain, slow the progression of painful neuropathy, and prevent it from developing in the first place.

Fit Feet

Neuropathy, combined with poor circulation, can lead to serious foot infections and deformities. When you cannot feel a minor foot injury, such as a bruise, burn, cut, or callous, and continue to use that foot, the injury becomes more severe. Furthermore, if there is inadequate blood flow to the injured area to aid in the healing process, an infection can develop easily. As the infection spreads into the underlying tissue and bone, portions of the foot succumb to cell death—a condition known as *gangrene*. Sometimes, the only way to keep gangrene from spreading is to amputate the infected body part.

Foot deformities often develop because the nerves that coordinate complex movements in the feet fail to do their job. We may put pressure on inappropriate (or injured) spots, thus causing further damage that then goes unnoticed because of a lack of pain sensation.

Each year more than seventy thousand people with diabetes require lower-limb amputations. Diabetes causes more amputations than all other causes combined, and loss of protective nerve sensation is the most critical factor. Even more disturbing is the fact that most people with diabetes die in less than three years after having a toe, foot, or limb amputated.

The good news is that tight blood sugar control helps to preserve healthy nerve function and blood flow to the feet. Lowering blood sugar levels also reduces the risk for infection. That's really good news for those looking to prevent foot problems as well as those recovering from existing foot ailments.

A Sound Mind

As we age, we're at risk for a number of health problems. Few instill as much fear as Alzheimer's disease, a progressive and fatal disease that destroys brain cells, thereby causing problems with memory, thinking, and behavior. Today, Alzheimer's is the sixth-leading cause of death in the United States, affecting more than five million Americans. Currently, there is no cure for the disease. Damaged blood vessels in the brain are believed to play a role in the development of Alzheimer's. Uncontrolled diabetes, which contributes to blood vessel damage, greatly increases the risk of developing the disease. *The good news* is that tight blood sugar control can reduce the risk of Alzheimer's to the nondiabetic population.

Flexible Joints

Joint mobility problems, including frozen shoulder, trigger fingers, and clawed hands, affect approximately 20 percent of people with diabetes. At the root of joint mobility problems is high blood sugar. Excess sugar sticks to collagen, a protein found in bones, cartilage, and connective tissue throughout the body. When collagen becomes sugarcoated, it thickens and stiffens, forming adhesions between adjoining muscles. This keeps joints from moving smoothly through the full range of motion. In addition to limiting movement, it can also cause pain in the joint.

The good news is that keeping blood sugar levels near normal reduces the risk of joint mobility problems. If you already have limited range of motion in your shoulders, hands, fingers, or any of your joints, lowering your blood sugar levels may help improve your range of motion and limit the pain associated with stiff joints.

A Positive Disposition

Blood sugar levels have a direct effect on mental well-being. People with diabetes commonly feel down when blood sugar levels are up. Depression is three times more common in adults with diabetes than it is in the general population. The mechanism of this increased risk is not entirely known. It could be related to the extra stress associated with living with a chronic illness, but because depression is often biochemical in nature, elevated sugar levels in the fluid surrounding the brain may also play a role. In addition, developing complications from diabetes can instill a feeling of helplessness, which is known to contribute to the onset of depression.

The good news is that improving your blood sugar can, in essence, make you a happier person. Researchers at the Harvard Medical School and the Joslin Diabetes Center studied the effects of blood sugar control on mood and disposition. They found that people with lower blood sugar levels reported a higher overall quality of life. Significantly better ratings were given in the areas of physical, emotional, and general health, as well as vitality.

So that's pretty much the situation. Blood sugar levels influence almost every aspect of our physical and mental well-being. Improving your blood sugar control will enable you to feel and perform better today as well as enjoy a longer, healthier life.

If you need a bit more motivation, there are countless examples of people with insulin-dependent diabetes who have achieved tremendous success in life:

> *Professional athletes* such as Jay Cutler (football), Catfish Hunter (baseball), Bobby Clarke (hockey), Chris Dudley (basketball), Bill Talbert (tennis), Michelle McGann (golf), Kris Freeman (skiing), and Gary Hall (swimming).
>
> *Entertainers* such as Mary Tyler Moore (the *Mary Tyler Moore Show*), Halle Berry (movie actress), Jean Smart (*Designing Women*), Zippora Karz (the New York City Ballet), and Bret Michaels (rock star).
>
> *Pioneers* Bill Davidson (cofounder of Harley Davidson), Thomas Edison (inventor), and Ernest Hemingway (author).
>
> Even former Miss America Nicole Johnson, former Miss Black USA Kalilah Allen-Harris, and former Mr. Universe Doug Burns.

Unfortunately, there are also people like my late father-in-law, a great man who succumbed to the complications of diabetes, and my wife's grandmother, who lost her legs, her eyesight, and eventually her life to poor diabetes control. So here's another "now" benefit of taking good care of yourself: peace of mind. There is something therapeutic about putting in a solid effort. Just knowing that you are doing your best can be a tremendous source of personal satisfaction.

There will be a cure for diabetes some day. It may not come in five years (like my doctor proclaimed twenty-five years ago), but when the day finally arrives, let's be in the best shape possible and not have any regrets.

Now let's get to work.

Chapter Highlights

- Managing diabetes takes work and sacrifice. There is no getting around that.
- There are many immediate benefits from managing diabetes, including physical and intellectual performance, emotional stability, safety, and well-being.
- The long-term complications of diabetes can be devastating, affecting virtually every part and system of the body.
- Tightening blood sugar control dramatically reduces the risk of developing long-term complications and dramatically slows the progression of existing complications.

3

Basics and Beyond

Managing diabetes is like building a home: Before you can even think about fancy fixtures and color schemes, you need to have a solid foundation. Prior to jumping into the intricacies of blood glucose regulation, let's take a few moments to get acquainted (or reacquainted) with some diabetes fundamentals. Even if you think you know all the basics, keep in mind that our knowledge of diabetes is constantly expanding. Here's your chance to get caught up on all the latest facts.

Diabetes by Any Other Name Is Just as Sweet

At the heart of our understanding of diabetes is the hormone insulin. Insulin's job is to facilitate the movement of nutrients—particularly glucose—out of the bloodstream and into the body's cells where they can be burned for energy. When not enough insulin is produced or the body's cells cannot use the insulin properly, blood sugar levels rise above normal and diabetes develops.

If you ask an endocrinologist to describe the different forms of diabetes, you'd better have some snacks handy because you're in for a long discussion. It's not just type 1 and type 2 anymore; many other forms of diabetes have been designated: gestational diabetes, LADA

(Latent Autoimmune Diabetes of Adulthood), MODY (Maturity On-set Diabetes of Youth), neonatal diabetes, and secondary diabetes. We'll get to those in a little bit.

In the vast majority of cases diabetes can be grouped into two major classes: the kind caused by loss of the ability to produce insulin and the kind whose underlying cause is insulin resistance (the body's inability to utilize insulin properly). Now here's where it gets interesting: People who lose the ability to produce insulin can sometimes develop insulin resistance, and those who have insulin resistance sometimes lose the ability to produce insulin.

Confused yet? Don't worry. You're not alone. Let's see if we can sort it all out.

All forms of diabetes cause blood sugar levels to be too high. Hypo-glycemia (low blood sugar) can also occur when insulin or insulin-enhancing medications (sulfonylureas or meglitinides) are used in the treatment. All require careful ongoing management, and all can pro-duce a wide range of health problems (complications). However, the similarities stop there. From a physiological standpoint, the various forms of diabetes and their modes of treatment vary like flavors of ice cream. First, let's look at the vanilla . . . er . . . type 1 diabetes.

Type 1 diabetes involves damage to the pancreas, a slimy organ nes-tled below the liver. At the base of the pancreas is a cluster of cells called the "islets of Langerhans" (named after the person who discov-ered them), and contained within the islets are "beta" cells. The beta cells are the cells that constantly measure blood glucose levels and produce insulin, as needed, to keep the blood sugar within a normal range. Along with insulin, beta cells secrete amylin, a hormone that, among other things, regulates the rate at which food digests.

In type 1 diabetes the body's own immune system destroys the beta cells. Normally, the immune system only attacks things that are not part of your own body, like viruses and bacteria. In an autoimmune disease such as diabetes, however, the immune system fails to recog-nize a part of your own body as such and attacks it. In the case of type 1 diabetes, the beta cells are attacked and destroyed over a period of months or years. As a result, the blood sugar level goes up and the body's cells are deprived of the sugar they need for energy.

> In type 1 diabetes, the body's own immune system destroys the insulin-producing beta cells.

There are more than one million people with type 1 diabetes in the United States, and several times that number worldwide. Tens of thousands are diagnosed with type 1 every year. Type 1 diabetes is usually diagnosed during childhood and adolescence, but it can also appear during adulthood. Most people with type 1 diabetes were born with an overactive immune system. We do not entirely understand what exactly triggers the attack on the beta cells of the pancreas. Viruses, major stress, environmental toxins, exposure to certain foods at a young age, and genetic markers have been proposed as potential triggers.

At the time of diagnosis a person with type 1 diabetes will likely have a very high blood sugar level and elevated ketones (acids formed from excessive fat metabolism coupled with insufficient sugar metabolism). Blood sugar levels above 180 mg/dl (10 mmol/l) also cause excessive urination, as the kidneys pass some of the sugar into the urine. In essence, high blood sugar causes you to urinate away many of the calories you consume. Consequently, rapid weight loss can occur. Frequent urination also makes you very thirsty. And because you are unable to get sugar into your cells without insulin, your energy level will be quite low and you will be hungry constantly.

Type 1 diabetes can be diagnosed a number of ways: through a blood sugar and urine ketone screening, by evaluating symptoms, or by testing for certain antibodies in the blood. Once type 1 is diagnosed, insulin treatment begins immediately. This initial treatment can provide a rest period for any beta cells that the immune system has yet to destroy. These remaining cells may be able to produce enough insulin to keep blood sugar levels relatively stable for a period of weeks, months, or possibly years. We refer to this as the "honeymoon phase" (or, more appropriately, "the calm before the storm"). Eventually, however, beta cell function ceases completely and insulin requirements go up and stay up. Without insulin, a person with type 1 diabetes will become severely ketotic (have high levels of acids in the blood), go into a coma, and die. This is the reason type 1 diabetes used to be called "insulin-dependent" diabetes: You depend on insulin to stay alive.

Approximately 90 percent of people with diabetes have *type 2 diabetes*. Type 2 is very different from type 1 in that there is no autoimmune attack, and the pancreas continues to produce insulin. In fact, for a while, the pancreas may actually produce more insulin than usual.

There are typically three stages to type 2 diabetes: onset of insulin resistance, followed by failure of the pancreas to meet the increased insulin need, followed by a reduction in pancreatic function. Let's look at these stages one at a time.

Stage 1: The Resistance

In order to do its job of taking sugar out of the bloodstream and packing it into the body's cells, insulin attaches to something called a "receptor" on the outer surface of the cell. This is similar to the way a key enters a lock in order to open a door. Once insulin attaches to the receptor, a "door" opens and sugar molecules are shuttled into the cell. So for insulin to work, there have to be sufficient receptors on the cell surface, and the insulin must find and properly fit into the receptors. *Insulin resistance* occurs when there are not enough receptors or the insulin has a hard time finding or fitting into them.

What causes insulin resistance? Typically, it is a combination of genetics (heredity) and lifestyle (the way we live). Having close relatives with type 2 diabetes greatly increases the risk. Certain ethnic groups, including Native Americans and people of African, Hispanic, Asian, and Pacific Island descent, are at a high risk. The aging process plays a role as well. The older we get, the more insulin resistant we tend to become.

Women who have polycystic ovarian syndrome (PCOS) often become insulin resistant due to the overproduction of hormones that oppose insulin's action. Likewise, hormones produced during pregnancy oppose insulin's action and can lead to gestational diabetes.

A lack of physical activity can cause insulin resistance in many people, as can stress hormones related to illness, surgery, or emotional turmoil. Steroid medications such as prednisone and cortisone also cause insulin resistance. But the most widespread reason people become insulin resistant is weight gain. Too much body fat, particularly around the middle, limits insulin's ability to function properly. In fact, gaining as little as ten pounds over a fifteen-year period can cause insulin resistance to double.

> The most common reason for people to become insulin resistant is weight gain, specifically too much fat around the middle.

Currently, more than forty-four million Americans are severely overweight. Obese individuals are *seven times* more likely to develop diabetes than those who maintain a healthy weight. And the problem is not restricted to adults: More than ever before, overweight children and teenagers are developing insulin resistance and type 2 diabetes.

Stage 2: The Production Shortfall

Insulin resistance affects a significant proportion of the worldwide population. Why, then, do only a fraction of those with insulin resistance develop type 2 diabetes? The answer lies in the resiliency of the pancreas.

When insulin resistance occurs, the pancreas needs to produce more insulin to keep blood sugar levels in a normal range. This is sort of like an office where one or two people aren't doing their job—everyone else has to pick up the slack. In most cases the pancreas can keep up with the added workload. But not everyone's pancreas has this capacity. If the insulin resistance becomes too much for the pancreas to overcome, blood sugar levels rise above normal. In other words, for type 2 diabetes to develop, you must have *both* insulin resistance *and* a limit to the pancreas's ability to secrete extra insulin.

To understand this concept better, imagine that you are an air conditioner trying to keep your house cool on a hot summer day. If you're one of those high-powered central air conditioning units that can crank out a bazillion BTUs, you'll have no problem overcoming the heat and keeping the house cool. But if you're one of those rusty window units, you're probably not going to be able to blow enough cold air to keep the house cool on really hot, humid days.

In this example, the heat and humidity are like insulin resistance: They present the challenge to the usual system. The air conditioner is like the pancreas: An efficient system can overcome almost any challenge, but a lesser system will be unable to meet the challenge. You need both very hot weather *and* a weak air conditioning system to create an oppressive situation.

At this early phase of type 2 diabetes, you can often achieve blood sugar control through exercise (which improves insulin sensitivity) and a healthy diet (which reduces the flow of sugar into the bloodstream). Sometimes you can use oral medications or noninsulin injectables to help the pancreas (or insulin) to work more effectively, and this may be all it takes. But it doesn't usually stay that way for long.

Stage 3: Function Reduction

Type 2 diabetes is a progressive illness. That is *not* a good thing. There is nothing hip, cool, or modern about it. It is progressive because it grows worse and becomes harder to control over time. After having diabetes for a number of years, insulin resistance tends to grow worse, and the pancreas struggles to keep up with the huge demand for insulin. Then a new problem sets in: Just like an air conditioner that is forced to run full blast every minute of every day, the pancreas starts to break down. (Heck, if you were asked to work day after day without any breaks and no end in sight, you would break down too . . . or at least find a new job!)

Two things cause the breakdown of the pancreas: overwork and a condition known as *glucose toxicity*. We can all understand the overwork part: Force those poor little beta cells into relentless slave labor, and many of them are going to die off. Glucose toxicity occurs when

high sugar levels do direct damage the pancreas, thereby further reducing its ability to produce insulin.

This is why the treatment for type 2 diabetes becomes more aggressive over time, and it explains why millions of people with type 2 diabetes take insulin injections—some once daily, some several times
each day. Does this mean that people with type 2 diabetes can eventually develop type 1? No, it does not. Remember, the type of diabetes is
defined by what *caused* it, not how it is treated. Type 1 diabetes occurs
when the body's own immune system destroys the part of the pancreas
that makes insulin. Type 2 is caused by insulin resistance, followed by
insufficient insulin production, which is followed by a gradual breakdown of the pancreas.

> The type of diabetes you have is defined by what
> *caused* it, not how it is treated.

If you don't currently take insulin for your type 2 diabetes but your
health care professional has encouraged you to do so, there is plenty
of good news. Insulin is the most potent and effective treatment for
elevated blood sugar. It is a more natural substance than pills (today's
insulin formulations are chemically similar to the insulin the body
produces), and lacks many of oral medications' side effects.

The fact is that oral diabetes medications and other injectables
have their limits. Unlike insulin, which lowers blood sugar *directly*, all
of the other medical treatments for diabetes work *indirectly*. This means
that they only work when the pancreas has the capability to produce
sufficient amounts of insulin and the body's cells are reasonably sensitive to the insulin. Once the pancreas is unable to keep up with the
workload, no amount of medication is going to solve the problem.

Taking insulin is easier and safer than ever before. The latest insulin formulations are much less likely to cause hypoglycemia (low
blood sugar) than are older types of insulin. Disposable insulin syringes have short, super-thin needles that you can barely feel. Insulin
can also be administered with prefilled pens: Simply dial up your dose

and inject. And best of all: When you begin using insulin and experience an immediate reduction in your blood sugar levels, you're probably going to feel better than you have in years!

The "Other" Diabeteses

Okay, I made that word up.

Remember, diabetes comes in more flavors than just vanilla (type 1) and chocolate (type 2). There are a host of exotic flavors to choose from.

Secondary diabetes (cookies and cream) involves destruction of the beta cells of the pancreas by something other than the body's own immune system. Potential causes include trauma (accidents/injuries), heavy doses of steroids, pancreatitis, alcoholism, cancer treatment, and infection. Regardless of the cause, the treatment is the same as with type 1: insulin, insulin, and more insulin.

Gestational diabetes (strawberry) is a temporary form of diabetes caused by insulin resistance that develops during pregnancy. Women with gestational diabetes usually require insulin to control their blood sugar levels. This is because oral medications pass through the placenta and may affect the baby's development. After delivery, when the production of insulin-opposing hormones drops off and weight comes down quickly, most of these new moms cease to need insulin injections. However, their risk for developing type 2 diabetes later in life is markedly increased. This is due to an underlying susceptibility to insulin resistance coupled with insufficient insulin production to overcome the resistance.

MODY (marshmallow) stands for maturity-onset diabetes of the young. Unlike type 2 diabetes, which is typically caused by insulin resistance, a genetic defect that limits the pancreas's ability to secrete sufficient amounts of insulin causes MODY. MODY is not associated with being overweight or obese. It is frequently diagnosed during early puberty, perhaps due to the increased demand for insulin that pubertal hormone production causes. Depending on how defective the beta cells become, oral medications or insulin may be required to treat MODY.

LADA (mint chocolate chip) refers to latent autoimmune diabetes of adulthood. Think of it as an incomplete, slowly developing form of type 1 diabetes that is compounded by mild to moderate insulin resistance. Some people call it "type 1½" because it shares characteristics with both type 1 and type 2. In LADA the immune system attacks the beta cells of the pancreas, but the attack is incomplete. Many beta cells survive and continue to secrete insulin, sometimes for years. Many people with LADA can manage their blood sugar with oral medications or low doses of insulin for a period of time, but eventually true insulin dependence develops and treatment requires intensive insulin therapy.

Neonatal diabetes (butter pecan) is a rare form of diabetes that occurs in the first six months of life. Similar to MODY, neonatal diabetes involves an inherited genetic mutation that limits the beta cells' ability to produce insulin. In some cases, neonatal diabetes disappears during infancy but then reappears later in life. In other cases, diabetes persists and remains permanent. Insulin is almost always required to treat neonatal diabetes and promote healthy growth and development.

Unlike the gazillions of books that explore the many treatment options for type 2 diabetes, this book focuses purely on the use of insulin. As such, it applies to everyone with type 1 diabetes, secondary diabetes, and neonatal diabetes, those in the later stages of LADA, as well as millions who suffer from type 2 diabetes, gestational diabetes, or MODY.

Table 3-1. Meet the Diabeteses

Diabetes Type	Cause(s)	Treatment Options
Type 1	Autoimmune attack on beta cells of the pancreas	Insulin
Type 2	Insulin resistance and progressive beta cell insufficiency	Lifestyle changes, diabetes medications, insulin
Gestational	Temporary insulin resistance	Lifestyle changes, insulin
LADA	Partial autoimmune attack on beta cells and some insulin resistance	Insulin, possibly diabetes medications in early stages
Neonatal	Genetic defect limiting beta cells' ability to make insulin	Insulin
MODY	Genetic defect limiting beta cells' ability to make insulin	Lifestyle changes, diabetes medications, insulin

The Gold Standard: Nondiabetes

To "think like a pancreas" is to come as close as possible to matching a normal, nondiabetic state.

Regardless of whether you have diabetes, blood sugar comes from two sources: internal and external. Internal sources are sugars that are stored up in the liver and, to a lesser extent, the muscles. External sources are the foods we eat—mainly carbohydrates. Our bodies convert internal and external sugar into a specific type of sugar called glucose for circulation in the bloodstream.

Glucose is the preferred energy source for most cells of the body. Some cells, such as brain cells and nerve cells, will burn only glucose for energy. Thus, having a steady supply of glucose available in the bloodstream is very important.

Insulin's job is to get glucose out of the bloodstream and into the body's cells so that it can be burned for energy. Besides helping get sugar out of the bloodstream and into the body's cells, insulin has another job: blocking the release of sugar from the liver and muscles. Instead, insulin packs sugar into the liver and muscles for use at another time.

When a person without diabetes has not eaten for a while, the blood sugar level can begin to drop. This can occur between meals, during sleep, and during exercise. When the blood sugar begins to drop, the pancreas decreases its production of insulin and increases its production of another hormone, glucagon. This reduces the amount of sugar being taken out of the bloodstream and stimulates the liver to release some of its stored-up sugar. As a result, blood sugar levels don't go too low.

In a way, the pancreas acts like a thermostat that keeps your house comfy-cozy. When the temperature goes up, the thermostat kicks on the fan and air conditioner. When the temperature goes down, the thermostat kicks on the heat. Either way, the temperature stays within a comfortable range.

In your body, when the blood sugar level begins to rise, the pancreas secretes extra insulin, which brings the blood sugar level down. When the blood sugar starts to dip a bit, the pancreas eases back on insulin production and begins producing glucagon, which brings the blood sugar back up. This system helps keep the blood sugar within a range that is comfy-cozy for your body—approximately 60 to 110 mg/dl (3.3–6.1 mmol/l).

Truth be known, a better title for this book would be *Think Like a Beta Cell*, because it is this select group of cells that acts like our blood sugar thermostat. (But who would want to read a book with that title? *Think Like a Pancreas* sounds much more fun!) In fact, the beta cells do more than just measure glucose levels and secrete insulin; along with insulin, they also secrete a second hormone called *amylin*. Amylin's job is to work with insulin, particularly at mealtimes, to keep blood sugar from spiking too high right after eating.

We will discuss amylin in more detail later. Let's turn now to the factors that affect our blood sugar levels on a daily basis.

Blood Sugar Balancing: The Major Players

There are a few major factors that affect our blood sugar on a regular basis (see Table 3-2) and a number of minor factors that pop up on special occasions (see Table 3-6 later in this chapter). Learning to keep them all in balance is what ultimately keeps the blood sugar under control. Let's start with the major factors.

Table 3-2. Major Factors Affecting Blood Sugar

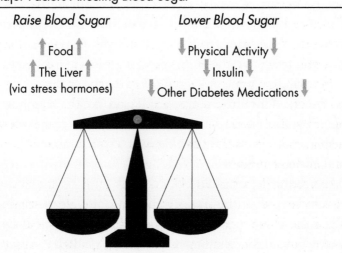

Raise Blood Sugar	Lower Blood Sugar
↑Food↑	↓Physical Activity↓
↑The Liver↑	↓Insulin↓
(via stress hormones)	↓Other Diabetes Medications↓

Factor 1: Insulin

Insulin lowers blood sugar, plain and simple. However, the action of insulin varies depending on the type of insulin, its rate of absorption into the bloodstream, and the body's sensitivity to the insulin.

Insulin is measured in units. A unit of insulin should lower the blood sugar the same amount no matter what kind of insulin you use. A unit of fast-acting insulin will lower your blood sugar the same as a unit of long-acting insulin; it just does so in a shorter period of time. One exception is a long-acting basal insulin called detemir (brand name Levemir), which is approximately 25 percent less potent than other insulins.

Another exception occurs when the insulin concentration varies. Worldwide, most insulin is standardized as "U-100." This means that there are 100 units of insulin in every cc (cubic centimeter) of fluid. In some instances, diluted (U-50) or concentrated (U-500) insulin can be found. Some people choose to dilute their insulin to allow dosing in more precise increments with standard insulin syringes. For example, a child who is very sensitive to insulin may have their insulin diluted to U-10 by mixing 90 units of neutral diluent with 10 units of insulin. The resulting mixture would be 10 percent as potent as normal U-100 insulin. One unit (as measured on an insulin syringe) would actually be equivalent to one-tenth of a unit of U-100 insulin.

A summary of insulin types is given below in Table 3-3. Be aware that the precise action times can vary from person to person. And because insulin is injected (or infused, in the case of an insulin pump) into the fat below the skin, the exact onset, peak, and duration can vary from day to day or even meal to meal.

Premixed insulins, such as 75/25 and 70/30, contain a combination of NPH (intermediate-acting insulin) and either regular or rapid-acting insulin. For example, Humalog Mix 75/25 contains 75 percent NPH and 25 percent Humalog. Novolin 70/30 contains 70 percent NPH and 30 percent regular insulin.

The actions of the newer insulins (lispro, aspart, glulisine, glargine, and detemir) are not affected much by where on the body they are injected, but older-generation insulins (regular, NPH) can vary considerably

Table 3-3. Insulin action profiles

Rapid-Acting Insulin *(lispro/Humalog, aspart/Novolog or Novorapid, glulisine/Apidra)*

Starts: 5–15 min   Peaks: ¾–1½ hrs   Lasts: 3–5 hrs

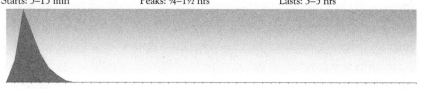

Short-Acting Insulin *(Regular)*

Starts: 15–30 min   Peaks: 2–3 hrs   Lasts: 4–6 hrs

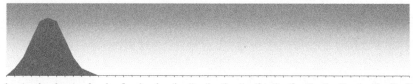

Intermediate-Acting Insulin *(NPH or Isophane)*

Starts: 1–2 hrs   Peaks: 4–8 hrs   Lasts: 12–18 hrs

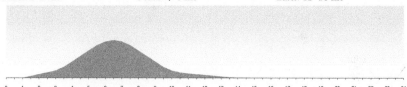

Long-Acting Basal Insulin *(detemir/Levemir)*

Starts: 1–3 hrs   Peaks: mildly, 6–12 hrs   Lasts: 18–24 hrs

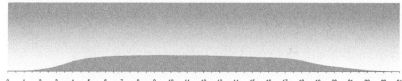

Long-Acting Basal Insulin *(glargine/Lantus)*

Starts: 1–3 hrs   Peaks: none   Lasts: 20–24 hrs

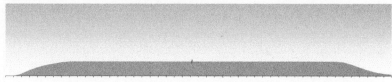

depending on where they are injected. However, injecting any insulin into a body part that will be exercising may accelerate the action of the insulin, particularly when the exercise is performed within an hour of the injection. This is due to enhanced blood flow in the area that is being exercised. For example, injecting insulin into the thigh and then going for a jog may cause the insulin to start working faster, peak earlier, and finish working sooner than usual.

Injecting insulin into muscle will also accelerate its action. Rapid-acting insulin, which normally takes three to five hours to finish working, can do its full work in ninety minutes or less when injected into muscle. This can cause a very rapid blood sugar drop, and it may produce hypoglycemia when given to cover a meal.

The action of NPH and regular insulin is more rapid in body parts that have greater blood flow. Injecting into the abdomen tends to produce the most rapid absorption, followed by the arms, then the legs, and finally the buttocks. When using older-generation insulins, be consistent about your injection sites. For example, always use the abdomen in the morning, thigh at dinner, and buttocks at bedtime. This will minimize the amount of variability in the insulin's action from day to day.

Below are a few other tips to help ensure that your insulin works as expected.

Rotate your sites: A condition known as *lipodystrophy* can affect insulin action. Repeated injections or infusions into the same small area of skin can cause the fat below the skin to either swell and harden (lipohypertrophy) or wear away (lipoatrophy). In either case, the absorption of insulin will be altered. For this reason, it is best to rotate your injection and infusion sites over a large area of skin. If it helps, imagine that you have a monthly calendar printed on each of the body parts where you inject, and inject into the spot that corresponds with the day of the month.

Storage: Unopened insulin vials, pens, and cartridges should be stored in a refrigerator (but not frozen). This should keep your insulin fresh until the expiration date. The butter compartment on the door might make an ideal home for your insulin. Once a vial, pen, or cartridge is opened (i.e., the rubber stopper is punctured), it may be kept at room temperature for up to one month. Room-temperature insulin tends to form fewer bubbles in the syringe and is generally more comfortable to inject. Your insulin should be kept out of direct sunlight and away from heating devices. When ordering insulin through the mail, request that it be shipped in a thermally insulated package. When traveling, keep your insulin in a cushioned pouch and do not leave it in a non–air conditioned vehicle for more than a few minutes. Do not use insulin that has an unusual appearance. If it has crystals on the surface, residue at the bottom, an unusual color, or if it does not mix uniformly, it should be discarded.

Replacement: As a general rule, insulin vials, pens, and cartridges should not be used for more than one month. Under special circumstances, such as when traveling extensively or if you forget to refill your insulin prescription, it may be used for slightly longer than a month. However, don't make a habit of it. Every time the rubber stopper is punctured, contaminants and impurities can find their way into your insulin and cause it to start losing potency. As a general policy, every month, discard whatever you have left and start fresh.

Proper mixing: NPH (cloudy) insulin, or any premixed insulin that contains NPH, needs to be rolled gently several times to ensure an even mixture prior to injection. NPH may be combined in the same syringe with regular or rapid-acting insulin. To ensure that your insulin is not contaminated during the mixing process, be sure to draw up the insulin in order from fastest to slowest. In other words, draw the clear (fast) insulin into your syringe before drawing in the cloudy (intermediate) insulin. If a tiny amount of fast-acting insulin gets into the vial of intermediate-acting insulin, it usually will not cause any harm. However, if intermediate-acting insulin gets into the vial of fast-acting insulin, it may contaminate the entire vial. Because of their slight acidic property, glargine (Lantus) and detemir (Levemir) should never be mixed with another insulin in the same syringe.

Spare the air: Whether you use syringes, pens, or a pump, eliminating large air bubbles is important. Very small (soda-sized) bubbles are not much of a concern, but larger bubbles can cause your insulin dose to be reduced significantly. Remember, room-temperature insulin is less likely to form bubbles. If air bubbles appear in your pen or syringe, you should inject them out through the needle (into the air) and then re-draw your dose.

The right depth: Because insulin is meant to be injected into the fatty layer below the skin, selecting a needle that is the proper length is important. A needle that goes too deep may accidentally inject into muscle. Not only does an intramuscular injection tend to sting, but any form of intermediate or long-acting/basal insulin that is injected into muscle can act much too fast and cause severe hypoglycemia. Likewise, injections that are too shallow (barely below the skin surface) can hurt and may "pocket" under the skin, resulting in incomplete absorption and high blood sugar.

Remarkably, skin thickness is similar in children and adults (even obese adults)—just a couple of millimeters. It is safe and advisable to use injection needles that are 4 to 8 mm in length. If only longer needles are available, try injecting at an angle in order to avoid accidental injection into muscle. For those who are very lean (including young children), pinch up the skin when inserting/injecting the needle. Release the pinch after injecting, and if using a pen, keep the pen needle in for five to ten seconds to ensure complete insulin delivery.

If leakage occurs after the injection (appearance of insulin on the skin's surface after removing the needle), consider leaving the needle in the skin longer or using a longer needle and injecting at an angle.

By the way, if the process of inserting the syringe, pen, or infusion set needle into your skin leaves you in a cold sweat, a number of injection aids are available. A list of such devices can be found in the Resources section in Chapter 10.

Factor 2: Other Diabetes Medications

Diabetes medications come in two forms: pills and injectables. Obviously, one of the injectables is insulin. But there are other injectables that can help to lower blood sugar, decrease appetite, and facilitate weight loss. We'll get to these later in this chapter. For now, let's explore the various oral medications.

Diabetes Pills

1. Pills that make you make more insulin
(only for type 2s, never for type 1s)

The original medications used to treat type 2 diabetes targeted the pancreas directly by increasing the production of insulin. This class of medications includes *sulfonylureas* (chlorpropamide, tolazamide, tolbutamide, glyburide, glipizide, and glimepiride) and *meglitinides* (repaglinide and nateglinide). Sulfonylureas work for twelve to twenty-four hours or more to lower blood sugar, whereas meglitinides work for only a few hours. Both sulfonylureas and meglitinides can cause hypoglycemia (low blood sugar) and weight gain.

Cut to the chase: Sulfonylureas and meglitinides are usually effective for lowering blood sugar levels in those who are in the very early stages of type 2 diabetes, before the pancreas has lost the ability to secrete sufficient amounts of insulin. However, by increasing the workload on the pancreas, these drugs may actually accelerate its breakdown. These drugs are of no practical use for people with type 1 diabetes or those with type 2 who have progressed to the point of requiring insulin injections.

2. Pills that slow the liver's sugar production
(mainly for type 2s, sometimes for type 1s)

The liver (the one in our bodies, not the one in the butcher's shop) is a major source of sugar that appears in the bloodstream. In most people with type 2 diabetes and many with type 1, the liver oversecretes glucose, making blood sugars harder to control. Since being introduced in 1994, the biguanide drug *metformin* has become the most widely prescribed medication for diabetes and one of the most widely used drugs in the world. Metformin decreases the amount of sugar the liver produces. Secondary benefits may include improvement in cholesterol levels and insulin sensitivity. Metformin is often used in combination with other diabetes drugs, including insulin. However, people with kidney impairment should not use it, and those with liver problems must use it with caution.

Cut to the chase: Metformin is often a drug of first choice for those with type 2 diabetes, and it may be beneficial to those with type 1 who require unusually large doses of insulin. Because the liver is mainly responsible for causing blood sugar to rise overnight, metformin can be particularly helpful to those with elevated fasting glucose levels.

3. Insulin sensitizers (mostly for type 2s, rarely for type 1s)

Thiazoladinediones (TZDs), including pioglitazone and rosiglitazone, are medications that increase the sensitivity of the body's muscle and fat cells to insulin. TZDs may be used in combination with other diabetes medications, including insulin. There is a risk of liver problems and fluid retention when using TZDs, so people with liver disease, poor heart function, or a history of congestive heart failure should not use them.

Cut to the chase: Those who are extremely obese but otherwise healthy can certainly benefit from the insulin-sensitizing effects of TZDs. The possibility of developing heart complications from TZD use has discouraged many people. And the fact remains that you can gain the same benefits TZDs offer simply by exercising and losing weight.

4. Digestion blockers (mostly for type 2s, rarely for type 1s)

Before being absorbed into the bloodstream, carbohydrates must be broken down into simple sugar molecules by enzymes in the small intestine. One of the enzymes involved in breaking down carbohydrates is called alpha glucosidase. By inhibiting this enzyme, carbohydrates are not broken down as efficiently and glucose absorption is delayed. When taken with meals, alpha-glucosidase inhibitors (acarbose and miglitol) tend to improve after-meal blood sugar control. However, because of the way they work, up to 75 percent of users experience abdominal pain, diarrhea, and gas.

Cut to the chase: Acarbose and miglitol may provide some help for those who experience blood sugar spikes after carbohydrate-rich meals. And because they don't cause hypoglycemia and may diminish between-meal appetite, they could aid those trying to lose weight. However, the side effects are more than most people are willing to endure.

5. Pancreas helper (mostly for type 2s, rarely for type 1s)

The newest of the diabetes medications, *DPP-4 inhibitors* (sitagliptin, saxagliptin), work by blocking an enzyme that breaks down a substance called GLP-1 (glucagon-like peptide 1). By increasing the amount of GLP-1 in circulation, DPP-4 inhibitors

- make it easier for the pancreas to release its stored-up insulin when blood sugar is elevated,
- decrease glucagon secretion from the pancreas,
- promote the growth and duplication of cells in the pancreas that produce insulin,
- slow the movement of food from the stomach into the intestines, and
- decrease appetite.

Sitagliptin and saxagliptin can be used in combination with other diabetes medications, but those with poor kidney function must use them very carefully. Although they have been proven effective for improving blood sugar levels without causing hypoglycemia, they have not been shown to reduce weight.

Cut to the chase: DPP-4 inhibitors offer multiple ways to improve glucose control with minimal side effects. They are the only oral diabetes medications that promote the growth and function of insulin-producing cells in the pancreas—a key to overcoming insulin resistance and managing blood sugar in type 2 diabetes.

Injectable Treatments for Diabetes

Until just five years ago the only injectable treatment for diabetes was insulin. Now we have three other injectables, with more on the way. Why the sudden upswing? As scientists learn more about how the human body actually regulates blood sugar levels, new and innovative treatments are unfolding before our very eyes.

1. Exenatide and liraglutide (mostly for type 2s, rarely for type 1s)

As mentioned earlier in our discussion of DPP-4 inhibitors, GLP-1 is a very important molecule in blood sugar regulation. Whenever we eat food that contains carbohydrates (sugar or starch), some of the sugar comes in contact with the inner lining of the small intestine. When this happens, cells of the intestine secrete special chemical messengers. One of these chemical messengers, glucagon-like peptide-1, or GLP-1 for short, helps the pancreas to release a rapid burst of insulin, decreases other hormones that raise blood sugar levels, slows digestion, and decreases appetite. Unlike insulin taken by injection or certain oral medications, GLP-1 does not promote low blood sugar or weight gain. Insulin secretion increases only when blood sugars are high and decreases as blood sugars approach normal.

Unlike DPP-IV inhibitors, which increase the amount of GLP-1 indirectly, exenatide and liraglutide, for all practical purposes, *are* GLP-1,

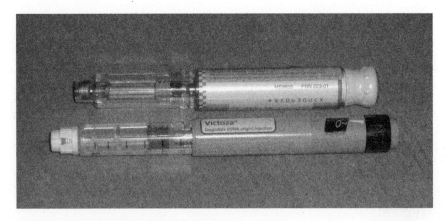

Pens for injecting Victoza and Byetta

except that they last much longer in the body than naturally occurring GLP-1. Currently, liraglutide (brand name Victoza) is a once-daily injectable, and exenatide (brand name Byetta) is taken twice daily, both via prefilled pens. Plans are under way to develop a form of exenatide that needs to be taken only once a week.

Because they require a functioning pancreas to work correctly, exenatide and liraglutide are intended mainly for people with type 2 diabetes. However, new research has shown that type 1s can benefit as well. Varying degrees of nausea are common during the first few weeks of usage, but this usually subsides over time. Those with gastrointestinal problems or kidney disease are usually not good candidates for either medication.

Cut to the chase: Despite having to be taken by injection and the short-term nausea that many users experience, exenatide and liraglutide have the potential to offset many of the factors that contribute to elevated blood sugar in type 2 diabetes. No other diabetes medication matches their ability to facilitate weight loss.

2. Pramlintide (for type 1s and type 2s who take mealtime insulin)

As mentioned previously, amylin is a hormone that the beta cells of the pancreas normally secretes along with insulin. People with type 1 diabetes secrete no amylin. Those with type 2 usually secrete insufficient amounts.

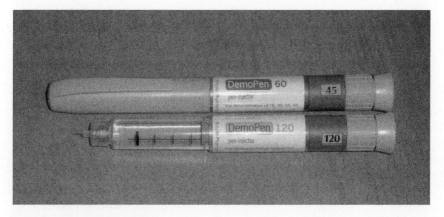

Pens for injecting Symlin

Classified as an "incretin" hormone because it affects the production of other hormones, amylin acts on the central nervous system to

- slow the emptying of the stomach's contents into the small intestine, where it is then absorbed into the bloodstream;
- blunt the secretion of glucagon by the pancreas (ironically, people with type 1 diabetes secrete extra glucagon right after meals); and
- decrease appetite.

By slowing digestion, reducing food intake, and minimizing glucagon production at mealtimes, amylin minimizes the blood glucose rise that occurs after meals. Postprandial spikes, as these are called, can influence one's energy level, intellect, emotions, and physical abilities. There is also growing evidence that spikes can raise the HbA1c and contribute to the development of long-term complications.

Pramlintide (brand name Symlin), the medication equivalent of the amylin hormone, is taken by injection via prefilled pen in fixed doses before meals. Due to its acidity, in its current form pramlintide cannot be mixed with insulin, and its effects only last a few hours. R&D specialists are working to develop a form of pramlintide that can be premixed with insulin, so someday the extra injections may not be necessary.

Besides aiding with postmeal blood sugar control, pramlintide can also be a valuable weight-loss tool. Users of pramlintide lose an average of six and a half pounds (three kilograms) over the first six months of use, mainly by consuming smaller portions at meals and snacking less often.

Pramlintide is intended for people who take insulin at mealtimes. Although not yet approved by the FDA for use by children, several studies have shown that pramlintide is safe and effective when adolescents use it in a supervised manner.

The most common side effect of pramlintide is nausea, typically twenty to forty minutes after injection. This usually dissipates entirely after a few weeks as the body becomes re-accustomed to having the amylin hormone present. Use of pramlintide has also been associated with an increased risk of hypoglycemia. Because digestion of carbohydrates is delayed when pramlintide is taken, insulin doses may need to be reduced and/or delayed as well.

Cut to the chase: Use of pramlintide certainly adds work and complexity to diabetes care, and the early side effects can be a detriment. However, postprandial (after-meal) glucose control continues to be a major challenge for most people who take mealtime insulin, and pramlintide has the potential to resolve this issue. And given that many people with type 1 and type 2 diabetes have difficulty controlling their appetite, adding pramlintide to one's treatment has obvious benefits in terms of lifestyle and weight control.

Factor 3: Food

Whoever said that there is no such thing as a free lunch really knew what they were talking about. Almost everything we eat or drink can cause blood sugar levels to rise.

The three major nutrients found in food are protein, fat, and carbohydrate. Protein's effect on blood sugar is minimal. One exception is when very little carbohydrate is consumed. Without dietary carbohydrate to provide glucose for meeting the body's energy needs, the liver begins to convert some dietary protein to glucose. For example, if you wake up to a breakfast of nothing but eggs and sausage, you may see a noticeable glucose rise a few hours later even though there was virtually no carbohydrate in the meal. However, when carbohydrate is present in a meal or snack, protein has little to no effect on the blood sugar.

Likewise, dietary fat's impact on blood sugar is usually of little significance. However, consumption of large amounts of fat can cause two distinct effects. First, it may slow the digestion of the carbohydrates that were consumed along with the fat, resulting in a slower, more gradual postmeal glucose rise. Second, large amounts of dietary fat, particularly saturated fat, can produce their own delayed rise in the blood sugar level several hours later. Here's how:

Step 1. You eat a high-fat meal or snack (this is the fun part).

Step 2. In a few hours the fat begins to digest; this continues for several more hours.

Step 3. The level of triglycerides in the bloodstream rises.

Step 4. High triglycerides in the bloodstream cause the liver to become resistant to insulin.

Step 5. When the liver is not responding well to insulin, it secretes more glucose than usual into the bloodstream.

Step 6. The blood glucose rises steadily as the liver's glucose output goes up.

For example, when having a heavy dinner at a restaurant, the carbohydrates may take a few hours to kick in due to fat slowing the digestion. Then, after you've gone to sleep the blood sugar may rise again through the night as the liver begins secreting more glucose than usual. But once again, these occurrences are reserved for situations when large quantities of fat are consumed. Small amounts of fat usually have no noticeable effect on the blood sugar.

> Large amounts of fat in a meal or snack may slow the digestion of carbohydrate and produce a secondary blood sugar rise after the carbohydrates have finished exerting their effects.

Carbohydrates are the nutrients that have the major effect on blood sugar levels. Carbohydrates (or carbs, for short) include simple sugars like glucose, sucrose (table sugar), fructose (fruit sugar), and lactose (milk sugar) as well as complex carbohydrates, better known as starches. Think of simple sugars as individual railroad cars, and starch as a whole bunch of cars linked together to make a train. Most starches are composed of many glucose molecules linked together.

Now here's the statement that has most people running to call their aunt who claims to know everything about everything. From the standpoint of blood sugar control, *whether the carbohydrates you eat are in the form of sugars or starches doesn't matter*. Both will raise the blood sugar by the same amount. A cup of rice containing forty-five grams of complex carbohydrate (starch) will raise the blood sugar just as much as a can of regular (nondiet) soda that contains forty-five grams of simple carbohydrate (sugar). And both will do it pretty fast.

You see, when you eat something that contains starch, the individual sugar molecules become unhooked from each other. This process takes place quickly, beginning the moment food comes in contact with saliva in the mouth. The individual sugar molecules start reaching the bloodstream within minutes—as soon as they pass through the stomach and reach the small intestine.

Table 3-4. Simple vs. complex carbohydrates

Foods rich in sugar (simple carbohydrates)	Foods rich in starch (complex carbohydrates)
fruit	potatoes
fruit juice	rice
raisins/dried fruit	noodles/pasta
regular soda	cereal
sports drinks	oatmeal
candy	bread
chocolate	crackers
cookies and cakes	bagels
pies and pastries	pizza
muffins	tortillas
milk	pancakes
ice cream	waffles
yogurt	beans
sport drinks	peas
table sugar	corn
honey	pretzels
syrup	chips
jelly	popcorn
beer	matzah

Also be aware that some "sugar-free" products can raise blood sugar. Having spent my first three years after college working in advertising, I can tell you that marketing people will do just about anything to get you to buy their products—even if that means bending the truth a little. "Sugar-free" can be put on a food label if the food does not contain sucrose (table sugar). However, a sugar-free food can contain complex carbohydrates, fructose (fruit sugar), and a variety of "sugar substitutes" such as sorbitol, xylitol, mannitol, lactitol, isomalt, and maltodextrin—all of which raise the blood sugar, albeit more slowly and to a lesser degree than ordinary carbohydrates do.

There are only a few artificial sweeteners that have no significant effect on blood sugar levels. These include saccharin, acesulfame K, sucralose, and aspartame. But once again, be careful. Products that contain these artificial sweeteners may also contain sugar substitutes or other carbohydrates that will raise your blood sugar level. The bottom line is that you should always read the label and make getting good at counting the grams of carbohydrate in your meals and snacks a priority.

We'll talk more about carb counting in the next chapter.

Factor 4: Physical Activity

Physical activity is a potent tool for lowering blood sugar. It does this by burning large amounts of glucose and improving the way insulin works, a process known as "insulin sensitization."

Think again about our door-and-lock analogy. Insulin is the key that opens up your cells, allowing sugar to ramble inside and get burned for energy. When you've been lying around like a sloth, your muscle cells aren't burning a lot of energy, so they only have a few doors available to open.

Now imagine that you temporarily lose your senses and decide to do your own gardening and landscaping work instead of paying a professional to do it. You. Yourself. With no real outdoor skills whatsoever (okay, I'm speaking from experience). All of a sudden, your muscle cells need lots more energy. As you begin accidentally mowing over the flowers that your wife painstakingly planted in the spring, the few doors that exist on your muscle cells don't allow the sugar to get in fast enough. The solution, as you might have guessed, is for your body's cells to make more doors and "grease the hinges." And that's just what happens.

Suddenly, those insulin keys find that opening the doors and shuttling sugar out of the bloodstream and into your cells is much easier, which gives you the energy to clean up the huge mess you created in the yard.

Unfortunately, nothing lasts forever. The extra doors your body's cells built are only temporary. After being sedentary for a day or more, the doors get taken down and you return to the way things were before your activity level increased. In fact, extended periods of inactivity can reduce your sensitivity to insulin, resulting in a state of insulin resistance. This, as you may have guessed, is a major characteristic of type 2 diabetes, but it can happen to people with type 1 as well.

As for burning glucose, the body burns almost exclusively sugar during the early phases of any form of exercise, and it continues to burn sugar throughout. Depending on your size and the nature of your physical activity, you might burn upward of 100 grams of glucose per hour! Below, in Table 3-5, is a general estimate of the amount of sugar utilized when you exercise:

Table 3-5. Glucose burned per sixty minutes of physical activity

	100 lbs (45 kg)	150 lbs (70 kg)	200 lbs (90 kg)	250 lbs (115 kg)	300 lbs (135 kg)
Low intensity	10–16 g	15–25 g	20–32 g	25–40 g	30–45 g
Moderate intensity	20–26 g	30–40 g	40–52 g	50–65 g	60–75 g
High intensity	30–36 g	45–55 g	60–72 g	75–90 g	90–110 g

But what's that? You've heard that blood sugar can go up during exercise? True, it can. But the physical activity is not what causes it. Physical activity always burns sugar and improves insulin sensitivity; maybe something else is going on at the same time, something we call a "stress response." This can take place during competitive activities, very high-intensity/short-duration exercises, judged performances, and sports that involve quick bursts of movement. To learn more about the stress response, see Factor 5 below.

Factor 5: Stress Hormones

Last weekend I decided to stay up late and watch a scary movie. It had something to do with super-gross vampires who get their jollies by eating the flesh of unsuspecting hotel guests. Anyway, after the final gut-wrenching, heart-pumping scene, I decided to check my blood sugar. And I'll be darned—it had *risen* about 200 mg/dl (11 mmol/l) during the movie. With blood that sweet, I felt like the grand prize for any vampires that might happen to be lurking in my neighborhood.

Earlier, I mentioned that the liver serves as a storehouse for glucose, keeping it in a concentrated form called *glycogen*. The liver breaks down small amounts of glycogen all the time, releasing glucose into the bloodstream to nourish the brain, nerves, heart, and other always-active organs.

The liver's release of glucose depends largely on the presence of certain hormones. Of all the hormones in the body, only insulin causes the liver to take sugar out of the bloodstream and store it in the form of glycogen. All the other hormones—including stress hormones, sex hormones, growth hormones, and glucagon—cause the liver to secrete glucose back into the bloodstream (see Figure 3-1 below).

Cortisol and growth hormone are produced in a twenty-four-hour cycle and are responsible for the blood sugar rise that we sometimes see during the night or in the early morning. The other stress hormones, particularly epinephrine (adrenaline), are produced when our

Figure 3-1. Hormonal effects on the liver's glucose secretion and storage

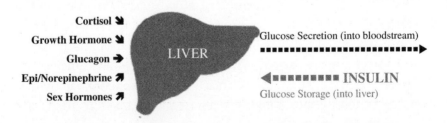

body needs a rapid influx of sugar for energy purposes. The glucose rise I experienced during the scary movie was no doubt the work of stress hormones.

Emotional stress (fear, anxiety, anger, excitement, tension) and physiological stress (illness, pain, infection, injury) cause the body to secrete a number of stress hormones into the bloodstream. For those without diabetes, an increase in insulin secretion follows the stress-induced blood sugar rise, so the blood sugar rise is modest and temporary. For those of us with diabetes, however, stress can cause a significant and prolonged increase in the blood sugar level.

The Little Stuff

If forgetting to recap the toothpaste or put the toilet seat down can wreck a marriage, imagine what the little things can do to your blood sugar!

Table 3-6. Secondary factors that can influence blood sugar levels

⬆ Tend to raise blood sugar ⬆	⬇ Tend to lower blood sugar ⬇
growth	alcohol
menstrual hormones	heat/humidity
later stages of pregnancy	heavy brain work
rebounds from hypoglycemia	previous intense exercise
gradual loss of beta cell function (type 2)	new/unusual surroundings
exiting the "honeymoon" period (type 1)	socializing
depression	stimulating environments
weight gain	early stages of pregnancy
excessive sleeping	beta blockers
caffeine	mao inhibitors
steroid medications	nicotine patches
diuretics	ritalin
estrogen	stress reduction
niacin	depression treatment

Little things do mean a lot. There are countless variables that can affect blood sugar levels—some raising it, some lowering it, and some . . . well . . . some seem to have a mind of their own. A number of these situations may occur on a semiregular basis, whereas others may happen once in a lifetime. Table 3-6 (on page 57) lists many such variables. We'll be spending the next several chapters focusing on ways to cope with and adjust to these variables in everyday life.

Chapter Highlights

- There are many forms of diabetes; the major ones are type 1 and type 2.
- Type 1 occurs when the immune system attacks the pancreas, destroying the insulin-producing cells.
- Type 2 begins as insulin resistance. If the pancreas can't produce enough insulin to overcome the insulin resistance, blood sugars rise. Later, the pancreas burns out, and as a result, more aggressive treatment is required.
- The major factors that raise blood sugar are carbohydrates and stress hormones.
- The major factors that lower blood sugar are insulin, diabetes medications, and exercise.

4

The Three Keys to Control

These days, everyone is talking about control. How's your control? Is your blood sugar under control? You don't want to get out of control!

Maybe it would be a good idea to define what we mean by "control." First off, I don't believe that diabetes should *control* anyone's life. There is much more to life than diabetes. If you're spending hours or more each day dealing with your diabetes, there is something wrong. Please, go smell the coffee . . . or the flowers . . . or something. In other words, as soon as diabetes management starts to get in the way of enjoying your life, it's time to ease up.

That said, I like to define quality diabetes control as achieving the lowest possible HbA1c without frequent or severe episodes of hypoglycemia and without your diabetes maintenance interfering too much with your daily life. Occasional, mild episodes of hypoglycemia are acceptable and not all that dangerous for most people. However, once low blood sugars become too frequent (more than two or three a week) or severe (causing accidents, seizures, or loss of consciousness), it will be in your best interest to control your blood sugar less intensively.

For those new to this diabetes management thing, *HbA1c* (also called a "glycosylated hemoglobin" or simply "A1c") is a laboratory blood test that provides an overall blood sugar average for the past

> Quality diabetes control means achieving the lowest possible HbA1c without frequent or severe hypoglycemia and without interfering too much with your quality of life.

two to three months (see Table 4-1 below). If you take insulin, getting an A1c test done every three months is a good idea. The A1c provides a more accurate average than you can obtain with typical premeal fingerstick readings because the A1c takes into account glucose levels all the time—before eating, after eating, while sleeping, exercising, watching TV, going to the bathroom, and so forth. An A1c that is much higher than expected (based on your usual premeal meter readings) may be a sign of after-meal or overnight high blood sugars. A lower-than-expected A1c could indicate that low blood sugars are occurring too often, possibly without any symptoms.

Table 4-1. HbA1c and average glucose

A1c (percent)	Avg. glucose (mg/dl)	Avg. glucose (mmol/l)
5	97	5.4
6	126	7.0
7	154	8.6
8	183	10.2
9	212	11.8
10	240	13.3
11	269	14.9
12	298	16.5
13	326	18.1
14	355	19.7
15+	Don't bother with numbers. It's high—real high.	

Technically, the A1c represents the percentage of red blood cells (the cells in our blood that carry oxygen) that have glucose stuck to them. When blood glucose levels are normal, approximately 4 to 6 percent of red blood cells will have glucose attached. Red blood cells live for an average of two to three months before they are broken apart and replaced with new ones. So, an A1c measurement gives us a good estimate of how high the blood glucose has been over the past two to three months. The formula for calculating your average glucose based on the A1c is in Table 4-2.

Table 4-2. Converting A1c into average glucose, and vice versa

Avg blood glucose (in mg/dl) = (A1c X 28.7)–46.7

Avg blood glucose (in mmol/l) = (A1c X 1.59)–2.59

and in reverse:

A1c = (avg blood glucose (in mg/dl) X 28.7)–46.7

A1c = (avg blood glucose (in mmol/l) X 1.59)–2.59

Why is A1c so important? The Diabetes Control and Complications Trial (DCCT) and United Kingdom Prospective Diabetes Study (UKPDS) showed that A1c is closely linked to the risk of both developing and worsening diabetic complications. Essentially, the higher the A1c, the greater the risk of developing and worsening eye, kidney, nerve, and heart problems. Given these risks, efforts should be made to keep the A1c reasonably close to normal. In most cases, that equates to an A1c in the 6 to 7 percent range. However, those who have hypoglycemia unawareness (don't receive low blood sugar warning symptoms) or significant heart disease as well as those who work in high-risk professions may seek slightly higher targets. Slightly higher targets are also reasonable for young children who cannot detect or treat hypoglycemia independently. Pregnant women, individuals planning for surgery, and those looking to slow or reverse existing complications may seek lower targets.

In any case, the goal is not simply the lowest average but also stability. Anyone can lower their A1c by taking too much insulin, but this would cause frequent and perhaps severe hypoglycemia. Instead, aim to achieve a good overall average with a high percentage of readings (or time, if you are using a continuous glucose monitor) within your acceptable target range.

Which begs the questions: "What should my target range be?" and "How often do I need to hit it?" Obviously, this is something that needs to be individualized and discussed with your health care team. With my clients, I recommend different targets for premeal versus the postmeal peak (one to one and a half hours after finishing eating). For the average person trying to achieve an A1c in the 6–7 percent range, a premeal range of 70–160 mg/dl (4–9 mmol/l) might be considered acceptable. Likewise, aiming to keep the postmeal peak below 180 mg/dl (10 mmol/l) is within reason. See Table 4-3 below for details.

Table 4-3. Acceptable pre- and postmeal glucose ranges

Level of control	A1c (percent)	Premeal acceptable range mg/dl (mmol/l)	Postmeal acceptable peak mg/dl (mmol/l)
very tight	5–6	60–140 (3.5–8)	<160 (<9)
tight	6–7	70–160 (4–9)	<180 (<10)
average	7–8	70–180 (4–10)	<200 (<11)
loose	8–9	80–200 (4.5–11)	<220 (<12)

This does not mean that you should expect to hit your premeal and postmeal targets every time you check your blood sugar. That would be like a baseball player getting a hit every time up to bat. What is reasonable is to get a "hit" at least 70 percent of the time, with fewer than 10 percent of your readings *below* your target range. This represents fairly stable control without excessive glucose swings. The degree of glucose variability can also be assessed by looking at the *standard deviation* of glucose values. This is a statistic that glucose meter and continuous glucose monitor download software can generate. We'll discuss this in more detail later in this chapter.

The Three Keys

Just as a chain is only as strong as its weakest link, successful diabetes management depends on three interlinked criteria: *tools, skills,* and *at-*

titude. Having one or two just won't cut it; all three are required. You could have the latest cutting-edge technology at your fingertips, but without the expertise to use it properly, it would go to waste. Likewise, fancy technology and top-notch skills fail to yield desired results without the ambition and desire to apply them properly.

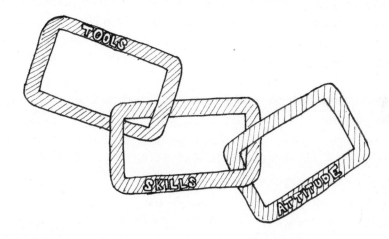

The Right Tools

Imagine trying to run the latest software on a computer built five years ago (maybe you don't have to imagine!). Likewise, trying to apply the latest diabetes management techniques with yesterday's technology can be equally challenging.

Below are some of the tools that make taking proper care of your diabetes possible.

The Latest Insulin

Today's insulin formulations are vastly superior to the insulins that were commonplace only ten years ago. (Of course, by the time *Think Like Your Entire Digestive System* goes to print, today's insulins may be equally obsolete.)

Yesterday's synthetic "human" insulins (regular, NPH, Lente, Ultralente) have been all but replaced by analog and basal insulins. Analog insulins (lispro, brand name Humalog; aspart, brand name Novolog or Novorapid; and glulisine, brand name Apidra) have a slightly different structure than regular insulin. This structural change allows the insulin to absorb much faster into the bloodstream, act more quickly, and match the blood sugar rise caused by carbohydrates better than regular insulin ever could.

Modern basal insulins (glargine, levemir) have chemical properties that make them activate in the bloodstream in a steady, gradual manner without a major peak—sort of like a time-released medication. This makes them much less likely to cause hypoglycemia than will intermediate-acting insulin (NPH). Not that NPH and regular insulin can't still play a role in diabetes management, but they certainly should not be the first choice for forming the foundation of your insulin program.

One other insulin option that is gaining popularity is U-500 regular insulin. As described in Chapter 3, U-500 is five times as concentrated as ordinary regular insulin. In other words, 5 units of U-500 has the blood sugar–lowering power of 25 units of regular insulin; 10 units has the power of 50 units. U-500 has become a popular choice among people who are extremely insulin resistant and require more than 300 units of insulin per day. The concentrated property of U-500 allows a person to take more manageable doses—a definite plus for those using an insulin pump or are limited by the size of standard insulin syringes. However, because U-500 acts even slower than regular insulin (its onset, peak, and duration take on the characteristics of NPH insulin), it should only be used in cases of extreme insulin resistance.

A Good Insulin Delivery Device

If you choose to administer insulin via injections, choose a device that permits the greatest accuracy as well as convenience and flexibility.

Disposable syringes are the traditional method for delivering insulin in the United States. (Most other industrialized countries have moved away from disposable syringes due to the large volume of medical waste they create.) When choosing insulin syringes, select the smallest size possible given your usual dose. This allows for the greatest dosage accuracy. Low-dose syringes are now available that have half-unit markings. If you rarely require more than 20 units in a single injection, choose

.3cc (30-unit) syringes with half-unit markings. If you sometimes require more than 20 units but rarely take more than 40 units in a single
injection, choose .5cc (50-unit) syringes. If you often require more than
40 units in a single injection, choose 1cc (100-unit) syringes.

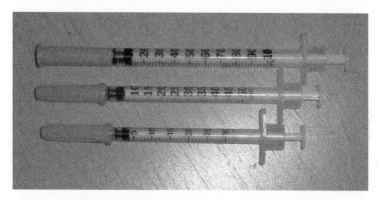

Choose the syringe size that meets your needs and permits the
most accurate dosing.

As far as the syringe needle, thinner is almost always better. Thin-
ness is measured by *gauge*. And here's where this gets interesting: The
higher the gauge, the thinner the needle (trust me, that wasn't my idea).
Make sure your syringe needles are at least 30-gauge. Depending on
your pharmacy or supplier, you may be able to get syringes with needles
that are as high as 32-gauge. As discussed earlier, the optimal needle
length depends on your body type, although needles longer than eight
millimeters are rarely necessary, even if you are very heavy. Using needles that are too thick or too long can cause unnecessary pain, bruising,
and accidental injection into muscle.

Insulin pens are discreet, safe, fast, and simple to use, making them
ideal for frequent meal/snacktime injections. Pens permit precise dosing by turning a dial on the top of the pen and then pressing a button
to deliver the insulin. In addition to visualizing the dose in the pen's
display window, the user can hear and feel clicks as the dial is turned.
Pens containing long-acting/basal insulin deliver in whole-unit increments. Pens that dispense rapid-acting insulin can administer either

whole- or half-unit increments. If you are fairly sensitive to insulin (i.e., if you take less than 25 total units per day), consider using a pen that delivers in half-units.

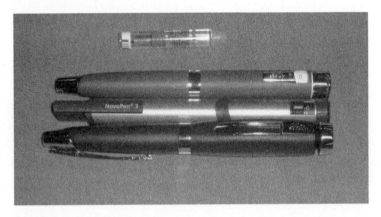

Durable pens use 300-unit disposable insulin cartridges. Some can deliver in half-unit increments.

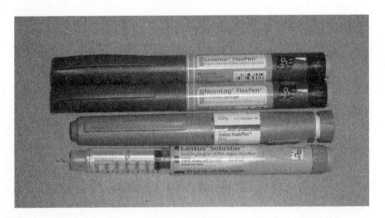

Disposable pens come prefilled with 300 units of insulin and deliver in whole-unit increments.

If you often require doses of one unit or less, a pen may not be your best option, as dosing accuracy is not as precise at doses that low. With any type of insulin pen, the pen needle must be kept in the skin for five to ten seconds following the injection in order to ensure complete and accurate insulin delivery.

Pens come either prefilled or with disposable insulin cartridges. The disposable needles used on insulin pens are thinner and sharper than traditional syringe needles, and hence they are more comfortable. Select a pen-needle length that is appropriate for your body type; four- to eight-millimeter needles should suit most people. A list of commonly available pens is located in Chapter 10.

Injection ports are an option for those with a significant dislike of frequent needlesticks. These devices (also listed in Chapter 10) require just one needlestick every two or three days in order to place a tiny, plastic infusion tube below the skin. Injections are given into a port that sits on the skin surface, so there is no skin puncture or discomfort whatsoever when insulin is injected into the port.

Needleless air infusers offer another option for those with severe needle phobia or allergies to the materials found in syringe and pen needles. Air infusers use pressurized air to create an insulin mist that travels through the pores of the skin at a high speed. When used properly, these devices can be virtually painless and may help to accelerate the action of mealtime insulin. Used improperly, however, they can cause bruising, scarring, and inaccurate insulin dosing. (See Chapter 10 for a listing of these devices.)

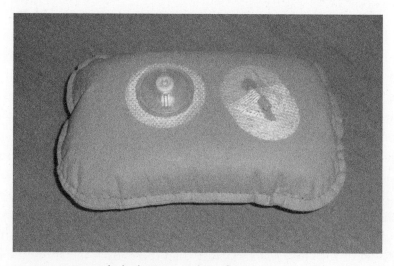

Injection ports include the iPro and Insuflon.

Insulin pumps were first developed in the 1970s, as scientists and physicians looked for a way to copy the world's best blood glucose control device: a healthy pancreas. The insulin pump mimics the pancreas by releasing small amounts of rapid-acting insulin (in tenths or hundredths of a unit) every few minutes. This is called basal insulin. When you eat, you program the pump to deliver a larger quantity of insulin fairly quickly. This is called bolus insulin.

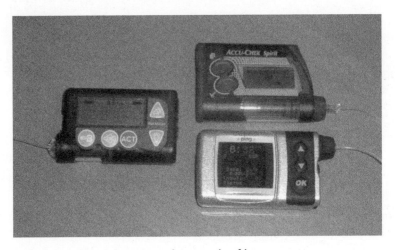

Today's insulin pumps are truly marvels of bio-engineering.

Insulin pumps are the size of beepers and contain a cartridge filled with rapid-acting insulin. They have a sensitive motor that turns very gradually to push insulin from the cartridge through a tube and into the body. Some of the newer pumps are referred to as "patch" pumps— the pump itself sticks directly to the skin and has its own built-in canula that infuses the insulin below the skin, so there is no tubing. Patch pumps are programmed via a remote control. It is important to note that insulin pumps do not control blood sugars automatically. It takes a skilled, educated, and motivated user to operate the pump properly and benefit to the fullest.

Those who use insulin pumps tend to have tighter glucose control with fewer lows and less variability than those using injections. Pump users also enjoy considerable schedule flexibility and report improve-

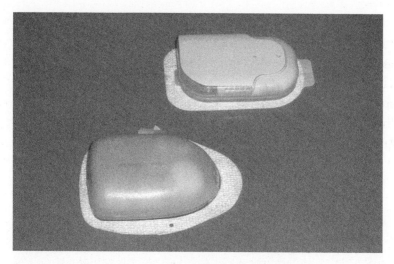

OmniPod and Solo are examples of "patch" pumps.

ments in overall quality of life. That's because, besides cutting down drastically on the number of needlesticks (usually one every three days), insulin pumps offer a number of unique therapeutic advantages over traditional injection therapy.

When using a pump, basal insulin delivery can vary by time of day to suit each individual's unique needs. You can make temporary adjustments to the basal rates for situations such as prolonged exercise, stress, and illness. In terms of mealtime and correction insulin (boluses), pumps have built-in bolus calculators that take your usual dosing formulas into account and deduct insulin that is still working from previous boluses. They can deliver with incredible precision—to the nearest tenth, twentieth, or fortieth of a unit. Pumps can also spread out the delivery of boluses over a period of time so that blood sugars don't drop after you consume slow-digesting foods. All pumps are downloadable and can provide considerable historical information for the user and their clinician.

Selecting a pump is a matter of personal preference. All pumps have a set of basic features that allow safe, precise delivery of basal and bolus insulin. Beyond that, a slew of buzzers and whistles, ranging from built-in bolus dose calculators to electronic links with meters and CGM devices, can be found. Shop around for the pump with the features you desire.

Besides the list of manufacturers and websites in the Resources section of this book, check out the thorough pump comparisons found at http://integrateddiabetes.com/p_compar.shtml.

In general, the features that are most important to consider when selecting a pump are as follows:

- Reservoir volume: Does it hold enough insulin to last you at least three days (the typical cycle for infusion-set changes)?
- Readability: Is the screen bright and sharp enough for you to read the details easily?
- Bolus amounts: Are the bolus increments (largest and smallest) suitable to your usual needs?
- Calculation features: Does the pump's bolus calculator allow you to enter your exact dosing formulas (insulin-to-carb ratios, target BGs, correction factors, duration of insulin action) without having to round off or compromise?
- Alarms: Can you hear or feel the alarms when they go off?
- Water resistance: Do you require a pump that is fully waterproof?
- Linkage: Do you want or need a pump that links electronically to a blood glucose meter or continuous glucose monitor?
- Wearability: Is the size of the pump and clip/attachment configured well for you?
- Coverage: Perhaps this is a good place to start. Check to see if your health insurance will only cover certain pumps or if the choice is yours.

Having a pump with the features you prefer can certainly make life more convenient, but as is the case with any instrument used to deliver insulin, achieving successful control has as much to do with the skills of the user as it does with the device.

Other Medications to Support the Insulin

Many people feel that just because they are taking insulin, all the other diabetes medications can't do them any good. Whether you have type 1 or type 2 diabetes, the other medications can make quite a difference.

For anyone who takes mealtime insulin and is experiencing after-meal blood sugar spikes, pramlintide (brand name Symlin) injections can provide significant improvement. As described in Chapter 3, Symlin can also help curb hunger for those trying to lose weight.

Metformin can also be used along with insulin. Because it blunts the liver's secretion of glucose into the bloodstream, metformin tablets can improve fasting blood sugar and reduce overall insulin requirements in people with either type 1 or type 2 diabetes, particularly those who are insulin resistant (requiring larger-than-normal doses).

For those who are highly insulin resistant, insulin sensitizing agents (thiazoladinediones) may provide some relief from very large insulin requirements. Just remember, though: If you have type 1 diabetes, none of these supplementary treatments will eliminate your need for insulin, but they may reduce the doses required to manage your diabetes.

A Modern Glucose Monitoring System

Without question, diabetes management requires frequent blood glucose monitoring. Trying to manage your diabetes without checking your blood sugar regularly is like driving a car with your eyes closed. You might be okay for a short while, but before long you're going to crash and burn.

The Blood Glucose Meter

Because you're likely to be checking quite often, look for a meter that is fast (some take as little as five seconds), simple to use (fewer steps means less chance for user error), downloadable to a computer (and with substantial memory), and easy on your blood supply (1 microliter or less is ideal; some require as little as .3 microliters). Many meters now are codeless, which means they don't require you to update the code number on the meter for each new vial of test strips.

The good news is that modern glucose meters are all reasonably accurate and unaffected by most over-the-counter medications. They also operate in wide temperature ranges and at varying altitudes. However, if you need to check your blood sugar under extreme environmental conditions, contact the various manufacturers (listed in Chapter 10) to find one that will work best.

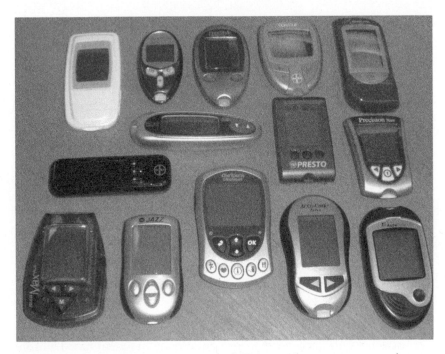

Most modern blood glucose meters are fast, compact, easy to use, and require very little blood.

Some meters have taken on the look and feel of minicomputers. Personally, I'm not a big fan of meters that allow entry of event markers and data such as insulin doses and carbs consumed because entering this type of information usually takes way too long and the data is displayed (either on screen or through a computer download) in a way that makes proper analysis difficult.

With the advent of meters that require very small blood samples, virtually painless alternate-site testing (taking blood samples from places other than the sensitive fingertips) has become a reality. However, be aware that alternate-site testing rarely works with meters that require one microliter of blood or more. Also, readings taken from the arm or leg may lag several minutes behind readings taken from the fingertips, so if you suspect that your blood sugar is dropping or rising quickly, a sample taken from the fingertip will provide a more accurate reading than will a sample taken from alternate sites.

Another feature that is new to some blood glucose meters is the ability to also check for *ketones* in a blood sample. The advantage of this system is that ketones will appear in the blood a few hours before they show up in the urine, and the meter provides a specific numerical value for the ketone level rather than simply small, moderate, or large. Abbott and Nova Biomedical make such meters. (See Chapter 10.)

Regardless of the meter you choose, having more than one is beneficial. Most meter companies will send you extra meters at no charge, assuming that you will continue to purchase and use their test strips. Personally, I keep a meter in each of the places where I am likely to do my testing—bedside, kitchen, desk at work, and gym bag. I don't keep one in the car because test strips can spoil easily at very high and low temperatures. Instead, I keep one in my briefcase for testing before I drive home from the office.

The Lancet

Oh, how far we've come since the "guillotine" days of yesteryear. Obtaining an adequate drop of blood with minimal discomfort is all about the tools and techniques you use. Lancets, like syringe needles, come in varying gauges. And like needles, the larger the gauge, the thinner (and less painful) the lancet. Look for 33-gauge (or larger) lancets. In fact, lancets as thin as 36-gauge are available for very young children. (See Chapter 10.)

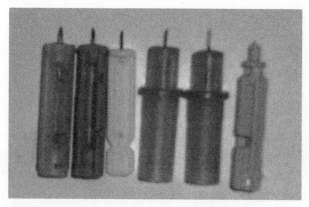

The lancet you choose *does* make a difference.

And whatever you do, *don't* just poke your finger with the lancet by hand. That virtually guarantees a painful fingerstick and buildup of scar tissue. Use a lancing device that has an adjustable depth setting. Start with the lowest/shallowest depth possible and see if you can conjure up a sufficient drop of blood with a little bit of "milking." If that doesn't work, go to the next setting and so on until you obtain a sufficient drop. That's the setting you should go with—and not a speck deeper. For alternate-site testing, it is best to use a lancing pen that has a clear cap (so that you can see when a sufficient drop appears) and a thinner head than those used on the fingertips.

Downloading Software

Virtually all modern blood glucose meters are downloadable to a PC running in a Windows operating system; many are also downloadable to a Mac if it has Windows-compatibility software. The meters themselves attach a time and date stamp to each glucose value so that you can generate graphs, charts, and statistics. Of course, it helps if the meter's clock and calendar are set properly, so check these before doing a download. (Nothing ticks me off more than doing a complete download and data analysis only to find that the a.m. and p.m. are backward!)

Meter downloading software is usually free of charge, available on the meter company's website or by obtaining the software on a CD. Download cables, which plug into your computer's USB port, are either free or modestly priced. Some connect directly to your meter; others use infrared or radio signals to communicate with your meter. We'll discuss what to do with the data obtained from your download in the Skills section later in this chapter.

A Continuous Glucose Monitor

Imagine buying a book that you've been dying to read and then only reading the first page of each chapter. Now imagine going to a movie that you've been dying to see and then spending 90 percent of your time in line at the concession stand, or listening to your favorite song through a broken headset that loses the connection every couple of seconds.

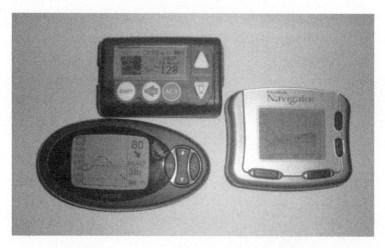

Continuous glucose monitors reveal the full story behind our blood sugar levels.

This is what life is like for those who only check blood glucose levels using a fingerstick meter a few times a day. We receive select bits of information, but we're missing the big picture—the full context of what is going on.

Now we can learn the full story. Continuous glucose monitors (CGMs) display updated information every couple minutes. They also provide trend graphs, warning alarms, and downloadable reports.

All of the currently available CGM systems utilize a thin filament inserted just below the skin to detect glucose in the interstitial fluid (fluid between fat cells). The information from the sensor is transmitted via radio signals to a handheld receiver, which displays an estimate of the current glucose level. Trend graphs, direction arrows, and high/low alerts are also provided. In some cases, the sensor information can be displayed right on an insulin pump. All CGM systems require occasional calibration by way of fingerstick readings. Even though they are not as precise as blood glucose meters (the sensors are generally within about 15 percent of fingerstick values), they still offer considerable value to the user.

One of the key benefits of CGM is the ability to detect *approaching* high or low glucose levels. Although they may not detect every high and

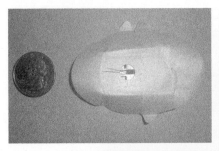
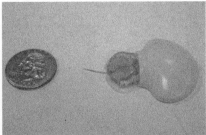
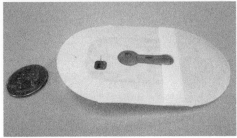

CGM sensors include a tiny filament that is inserted just below the skin as well as an attachable radio transmitter.

low, CGMs provide an early warning for the vast majority—and much earlier than most people can feel them on their own. The trend arrows/ graphs give us the ability to forecast where the glucose is headed so that appropriate decisions can be made regarding food, activity, and insulin/ medication. For example, you would probably act differently if you knew that a bedtime reading was 100 mg/dl (5.5 mmol/l) and dropping quickly as opposed to the same value but steady.

All CGM receivers are downloadable for analyzing overall statistics and trends. The downloaded data can be used to measure the magnitude of postmeal spikes, test the effectiveness of basal insulin, evaluate postmeal and postexercise patterns, detect nighttime lows or rebounds, and measure the precise action curve for rapid-acting insulin. Research has shown that those who use their CGM consistently tend to have fewer (and less severe) lows and improvements in their A1c, along with less variability in their glucose levels. Those who don't use them on a consistent basis may benefit while wearing them but tend to see little in terms of long-term improvements.

Why would anyone *not* use a CGM all the time? Well, they do have a few drawbacks. Inserting the sensor can be a bit awkward and uncomfortable, and having something stuck on the skin all the time bothers some people. There are periods of inaccuracy and occasional false alarms, and there is inherent lag time in any CGM system (their readings lag about ten minutes behind actual blood glucose values). Many people prefer not to carry around the receiver wherever they go. However, there is a growing movement toward linking the sensors and transmitters with devices such as insulin pumps, smart phones, and other common handheld devices.

And finally, there are costs: Even with insurance coverage, there are usually copays and deductibles that you must meet.

To know if CGM is right for you, especially without trying one first, is difficult. Insurance coverage for the systems and disposable sensors has improved considerably over the past few years. The CGM companies all offer a thirty-day return policy, so, from that standpoint, there is little risk. My practice (Integrated Diabetes Services) also provides CGM system trials for one to two weeks, with follow-up analysis of the data.

So before dismissing the whole idea, remember this: When home blood glucose meters first came out, many people were skeptical of them as well!

A Supportive Health Care Team

We've all heard the saying, "A lawyer who defends himself has an idiot for a client." The same holds true for anyone who neglects to call on the expertise of health care professionals for proper diabetes care.

Surrounding yourself with a quality health care team is like putting together a winning basketball team. Each player has a role, yet all should work collaboratively for your benefit. Your job is to assemble the team and hold them accountable for doing their jobs. That means you may have to fire or trade some players from time to time, but that's okay. Unless you're winning championships every year, getting a fresh perspective once in a while helps.

One approach is to go with a preassembled team of diabetes professionals. The American Diabetes Association keeps a list of "recognized diabetes self-management programs," most of which feature a multi-disciplinary group of diabetes-care specialists. Although there are many quality providers not included on the list, the American Diabetes Association has recognized all the programs on the list for meeting national standards for diabetes education and treatment. For an updated list go to http://professional.diabetes.org/erp_list.aspx, or call 800-342-2383.

Otherwise, look for the following to create your own team of diabetes health care all-stars:

A certified diabetes educator. A CDE is often a nurse or dietitian, but he or she can also be a pharmacist, exercise physiologist, physician, mental health counselor, or anyone in the health care field with advanced training in diabetes management. Your CDE should be able to coach you through the complexities of living day to day with diabetes. CDEs are expert teachers as well as skilled clinicians. If you can find a CDE (or physician) who also has diabetes, you can tap into a gold mine of both personal and professional experience. To locate a CDE in your area, talk to your doctor or visit the American Association of Diabetes Educators' CDE network at http://www.diabeteseducator.org/Diabetes Education/Find.html. My practice provides the services of skilled CDEs with a direct personal link to diabetes via phone and the Internet as well as in person. Visit www.integrateddiabetes.com, or call 877-735-3648 for information.

A physician. Different physicians have different levels of expertise in treating diabetes. *Endocrinologists* typically have the most experience and skill in diabetes care. However, some endocrinologists specialize in treating other endocrine disorders (e.g., pituitary or thyroid problems) or are more adept at treating non-insulin-using type 2s than those who utilize intensive insulin therapy. Internal medicine doctors (internists) usually treat a variety of chronic health conditions, diabetes being just one of them. Some internists have a great deal of expertise in treating diabetes; others tend to refer their insulin-using patients elsewhere. General practitioners (family doctors) typically treat many short- and long-term illnesses and have only a basic understanding of how to manage diabetes.

Look for a physician who is board certified; this ensures that they receive continuing education and are updated on the latest treatment methods. To find a board-certified physician, visit the American Board of Medical Specialties website at www.abms.org. Regardless of the type of physician you hire, he or she is ultimately responsible for screening for complications, prescribing the necessary tests and medications, intervening in case of a crisis, keeping you abreast of the latest developments in diabetes care, and making sure that your control is on track. If your physician is not meeting these minimum criteria, fails to answer your questions to your satisfaction, or does not support your pursuit of new technologies, management approaches, or other health care specialists, consider looking for someone else.

A registered dietitian. Given the heavy influence that food has on diabetes control, it pays to have a nutrition expert in your corner. An RD can work with you to increase your knowledge and skills in carbohydrate counting, weight control, sports nutrition, special occasion dining, vegetarian meal planning, alcohol safety, and dietary management of conditions such as hypertension, gluten intolerance, and elevated cholesterol. To find an RD who specializes in diabetes, contact the American Dietetic Association at 800-877-1600, or visit www.eatright .org/public (click on the "find a nutrition professional" icon).

A mental health counselor. With all the pressure placed on people with diabetes to manage blood sugar levels while still taking care of everything else life throws at us, a mental health counselor can be a valuable member of your health care team. Mental health professionals—social workers, psychologists, and psychiatrists—can help with issues such as stress, depression, eating disorders, sleep disturbances, obsessive/compulsive behaviors, anxieties, relationship difficulties, financial hardship, and job discrimination. In most cases, psychological issues must be dealt with before you can do an effective job managing your diabetes. So if you are experiencing issues that may be interfering with your ability to take proper care of yourself, don't hesitate to ask your physician for a referral to a mental health professional.

The exercise specialist. Exercise remains a hot topic in diabetes because of all the benefits it has to offer. However, you can also get yourself in hot water if you exercise improperly. Severe hypoglycemia, acute injuries, and worsening of diabetic complications are among the risks that people with diabetes who exercise face. An exercise physiologist is a health professional who understands the physical, psychological, and metabolic effects of exercise. He or she can help you design an exercise plan, formulate strategies to prevent hypoglycemia, manage blood sugars during sports/competitive activities, and reduce your risk for injuries and other complications. Look for an exercise physiologist who is also a diabetes educator; many ADA-recognized diabetes centers and programs affiliated with large medical institutions offer the services of exercise physiologists.

Specialists. Given the complexity of diabetes and the many organ systems that are affected, adding a few other specialists to your health team would be wise. These include:

- podiatrist (for preventive foot care and treatment of foot problems)
- ophthalmologist (for routine eye exams and treatment of eye disorders)
- dentist (for ongoing tooth/gum care and treatment of periodontal disease)
- nephrologist (for treatment of kidney disorders)
- neurologist (for treatment of nerve disorders)
- cardiologist or vascular surgeon (for treatment of large blood vessel diseases)

The Right Skills

Modern technology is useless without the know-how to utilize it properly. Take my wife (please . . . and please don't show her this!). Her computer at work is equipped with a powerful processor and all the latest software, but she prefers to use it as a place to tack up her sticky notes. Likewise, high-tech diabetes management devices are nice, but ultimately, your skill is what gets you the control you want.

The following are skills that everyone using insulin should adopt.

Self-Monitoring

From my experience, people who check their blood sugar levels four to eight times daily tend to have the best overall control. Checking less frequently is like taking your hands off the steering wheel while driving: You might stay on the road for a few moments, but before long you are going to veer into dangerous places. Frequent checks allow you to detect (and fix) high glucose levels so that you don't go for long stretches above your target range. They also give you a chance to detect (and fix) dropping glucose levels *before* hypoglycemia develops. However, too much of a good thing may not be so good. Checking obsessively (e.g., every hour of every day) may actually do more harm than good. Besides creating unhealthy dependence and anxiety, it may cause you to overreact to mild highs or lows before your insulin (or your food) has a chance to take effect. And remember one of our requirements for quality diabetes control: Managing your diabetes should *not* get in the way of enjoying the rest of your life.

In general, the best times to check blood sugars are

- before each meal and snack (to determine if a correction dose is needed and to evaluate the effectiveness of the previous dose);
- prior to exercise and driving (particularly if a reading has not been taken recently);
- periodically, one hour after meals (to assess postmeal control);
- before going to sleep; and
- periodically, in the middle of the night (to verify that your basal insulin is holding you steady while you sleep).

To help ensure the accuracy of your readings, be sure to use test strips prior to their expiration date. Keep the strips sealed in their bottle or foil wrapping, and be sure to apply enough blood to cover or fill the test area completely. Never expose your strips to extreme hot or cold temperatures—so don't leave them in your car. If your meter requires coding, make certain that the code number in the meter matches the code number on the test strip packaging.

A clean finger is also a must. There is no need to wipe your finger with alcohol, but the presence of dirt, grease, food, or other foreign substances on your finger can affect the accuracy of the reading. Last week I had an opportunity to try some of the finest barbecue Kansas City has to offer. After devouring a few ribs, I checked my blood sugar and was very surprised to see a reading of 438 mg/dl (24 mmol/l). After cleaning my finger and rechecking, the reading was 108 (6)—quite a difference. At that point, two thoughts crossed my mind: I'm glad I didn't take insulin for the high reading, and *man, that's some powerful sauce!* If you ever suspect that your meter reading may be inaccurate, recheck—twice if necessary. If you're still in doubt, use the "control solution" that came with your meter to verify its accuracy. The reading obtained with the control solution should fall within the designated range on the test strip package. If the result is outside of the reference range, try a new package of strips. If that does not solve the problem, call the meter manufacturer and ask for a replacement meter.

'Self-monitoring also means checking your HbA1c about every three months. This will keep you accountable and provide feedback regarding the effectiveness of your current program. Many diabetes clinics can perform A1c tests using a simple fingerstick procedure. One-time-use home A1c kits are also available. (See Chapter 10.)

A few other measures of long-term glucose control are also available. A *glycosylated fructosamine* test assesses glucose control over the past two to three weeks. This lab test can be used if you have blood abnormalities that may interfere with the accuracy of an A1c. It can also be used if you need to maintain very tight control for special situations such as pregnancy or preparation for surgery. Another test, the GlycoMark, evaluates the degree to which blood glucose levels spike after meals. It evaluates how often (and how much) glucose levels are above the renal threshold, which is usually 160–180 mg/dl (9–10 mmol/l) over a one- to two-week period. This test can be useful if your A1c is much higher than your premeal fingerstick readings would indicate. Strategies for managing after-meal spikes are covered in Chapter 9.

Record Keeping

It's a fact: People who keep written records have better glucose control than those who don't. Of course, you could say that those who keep records do so because their numbers look good on paper, but you can't deny that keeping records makes us feel accountable for our actions, and maintaining organized, detailed records and analyzing them on a regular basis allows us to catch problems and fine-tune more easily.

Any good record-keeping system begins with blood glucose readings. For those taking only basal insulin (once or twice daily), blood sugar readings should be taken twice daily—at least while control is being fine-tuned. Ideally, the readings should be taken at two meals in a row and rotated from day to day. For example, on day one, test before breakfast and lunch. On day two, test before lunch and dinner. On day three, test at dinner and bedtime. Then repeat the process from day one. This approach lets you see when blood sugar levels may be rising or falling.

For those taking basal as well as mealtime insulin (or two injections of premixed insulin daily), blood sugar should be checked a minimum of four times daily—upon waking, midday, predinner, and at bedtime.

Blood sugar readings by themselves are not of much use unless they are all running high or low. For most of us, however, that just isn't the case. When inconsistencies exist, you need to figure out *why* the readings went high or low. Were they caused by too much or too little food? Incorrect insulin doses? Changes in physical activity? Stress or illness?

To figure out why your blood sugar levels vary, record the amount of insulin taken; the grams of carbohydrate consumed at each meal and snack; the type and length of exercise and other physical activities performed, including housework, yard work, shopping, and extended walking; as well as stresses that tend to affect blood sugars (e.g., illness, menstrual cycles, emotional events, and hypoglycemic episodes). Pump users should also note when infusion set changes take place.

To get the most from your record keeping, organize the information so that it will be easy to analyze. Forms like those in Appendix A have been very helpful to my patients. These forms are also available at my website in a printable and downloadable form, http://www.integrated diabetes.com/logs.shtml.

If you're sitting there saying, "No need. I can just download my thingamabob to the computer. It keeps all the information for me." Sorry, bud. At this point there is no good replacement for a written record-keeping system. Downloadable devices and electronic databases fail to capture many of the key events that influence our blood sugar levels, and none present the information in a format that is practical to analyze. So at least for the time being, get out the pen and paper, or save the forms from our website to your computer and type the data in. Do you need to do it forever? Probably not. I find that once the insulin doses have been properly fine-tuned, written record keeping can be done periodically (perhaps one week per month) or any time blood sugars are starting to fall outside of your desired range. Of course, some people take comfort in keeping ongoing records, feeling that it keeps them on track. If you're one of those people, then keep on loggin'!

> At this point, there is no good replacement for an organized written record-keeping system.

Data Analysis

Learning how to interpret your self-monitoring records is also essential. Otherwise, your log sheets are nothing more than pieces of paper with a bunch of numbers and little blood spots on them.

Review your own records on a weekly or bimonthly basis. Keep track of how many readings are above, below, and within your target range for each time of day that you test. If more than 25 percent of your readings are above target, or more than 10 percent are below your acceptable range, changes to your insulin program or dosing formulas may be in order. Because low blood sugars can sometimes produce high readings a few hours later, eliminating the lows before addressing the highs is usually the best course of action.

Besides evaluating your blood glucose levels by time of day, see if you can detect what may be causing the highs and lows. Here are some questions to ask yourself:

- Are the patterns different on certain days of the week? Certain phases of the month?
- Is physical activity having an immediate or delayed effect?
- Do certain types of foods always seem to make your blood sugar rise?
- Are you always high after experiencing a low? Or do lows tend to repeat themselves?
- Are you often low (or still a bit high) after taking extra insulin for a high reading?
- Are emotional situations impacting your control?
- Does your control vary based on how long you have used an insulin pen, vial, or pump infusion set?

When it comes to reducing the frequency of the highs and lows, the culprit is not always one of the "usual suspects." One of my clients, a curbside baggage handler at the airport, discovered that how much luggage he processed greatly influenced his daytime blood sugar. On the busiest travel days—Fridays and Sundays—his blood sugars were much lower than the rest of the week. A simple reduction in his meal-time insulin on busy days solved the problem.

Another client had nice, consistent readings except for highs on certain evenings. A look at her logbook showed that choir practice usually preceded her high blood sugars. It seems that the passion and emotion she felt while singing were causing an adrenaline-induced rise in her blood sugar. A little extra insulin before practice solved the problem nicely.

One of our young clients, a second grader using a bright pink insulin pump, had very erratic readings when reporting to the nurse before lunch—some highs, some lows, but rarely on target. Her records revealed that the lows were on days she had gym class in the morning, and the highs were on nongym days. A slight tweaking of her morning insulin based on her level of activity put her blood sugars back on track.

Remember, managing diabetes isn't about achieving instant perfection; rather, it's about making improvements. Every time you make a sensible adjustment based on your records, your control should get just a little bit better.

Analyzing Meter, Pump, and CGM Downloads

When written records are not available, electronic devices such as blood glucose meters, insulin pumps, and continuous glucose monitors can provide useful information, *if* you know what to look for. Beautiful pies and bars (charts) are better suited for eating than insightful data analysis. The information and reports that can yield valuable insight include the following:

Statistics

When viewing data over the past couple of weeks or more, focus on the overall average glucose, standard deviations, and percentage of readings that are above, below, and within your target range. The average should correlate well with your HbA1c, although it may underestimate a bit if you don't do much after-meal testing (BGs tend to spike up for a short while after meals and snacks).

The standard deviation (SD) reflects the amount of *variability* in your readings. Lower is better. If the SD is more than half of your average, your readings include many extreme highs and/or lows. An SD that is less than one-third of your average means that your readings are fairly consistent from day to day, without too many in the extreme ranges.

The percent of readings (or time) within your target range is the gold standard for assessing the quality of your diabetes management. Though a couple of extreme highs or lows can greatly influence your average and SD, they won't necessarily wreck your percent in-range. In your software be sure to set *your* target range (the default setting is often unrealistic).

The percent of readings in-range (or time spent in range) is the gold standard for assessing the quality of your diabetes control.

In some meter and pump software packages more detailed statistics are sometimes available. These include averages by day of the week (to see if you are having control issues related to your weekly schedule) and averages and percent high/low/in-range by mealtime.

Downloads of continuous glucose monitors offer another level of statistical information: percentage of actual time spent above, below, and within your target range; area under the curve (AUC), which reflects the time and magnitude of above-range glucose levels; cumulative average glucose, which should correlate closely with HbA1c; and the number of excursions above and below your target range.

Modal (or Standard) Day Reports

This report provides a scatter plot of blood glucose values arranged by time of day. It serves as a quick visual summary of the *quality* of your blood glucose control, grouped according to your usual mealtimes. (See Figure 4-1 below.) As was the case with setting your target BG range, be

Figure 4-1. Example of a modal day report

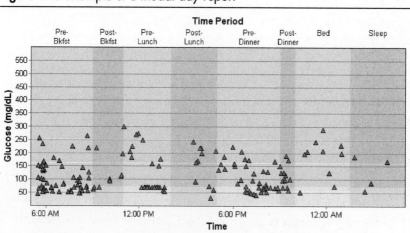

sure the meal schedule in the software corresponds with *your* usual schedule. (Many are preset for the "early bird special" crowd, with meals and bedtime at very early times of day.)

Take a look at your modal day report for the past several weeks. Are there frequent highs or lows at certain times of day? Are the readings consistent or widely scattered? When you view it in conjunction with the averages and percent high/low/in-range statistics described above, you will have a very nice overview of your daily control.

Sensor Overlay Reports

CGM download software can superimpose multiple days of sensor data onto a single report. (See Figures 4-2 and 4-3 below.) This report reveals unique insight into the glucose ebb and flow on a typical day, helping you answer questions such as:

- When are most highs and lows occurring?
- Are glucose levels peaking very high after certain meals?
- Is there an upward or downward trend overnight?
- Do lows trigger rebound highs?
- How long does it take for bolus insulin to finish working?
- Are lows occurring without warning signs or symptoms?

Figure 4-2. Example of a sensor overlay report

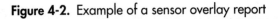
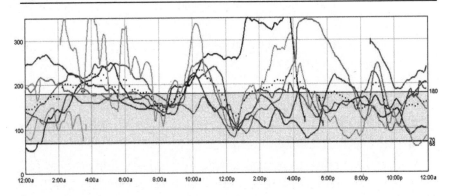

Figure 4-3. Example of a sensor overlay report

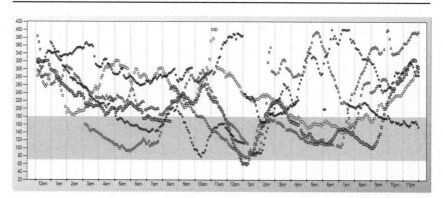

Logbook Report

Summary statistics (averages, SD, percent in-range) and modal day reports can be misleading if you check more than once when your blood glucose is high or low or if you tend to check more often when you feel that something isn't quite right. The logbook report permits a more accurate assessment of your blood glucose history, listing readings in chart form according to the time of day. Once again, be sure to set up the software so that the time intervals correspond with your typical schedule.

A detailed look at your logbook can answer questions such as:

- Do lows tend to occur after highs? (Perhaps you are overdosing for the highs.)
- Do highs tend to occur after lows? (Perhaps you are overeating or rebounding.)
- Do you tend to run several highs in a row? (Perhaps your correction doses are insufficient.)
- Do glucose levels change overnight or between meals? (Perhaps your basal insulin needs adjustment.)
- Are there patterns related to when you do—or don't—exercise?
- Are there patterns after you eat restaurant or take-out food?

Glucose Trend Graphs

Trend graphs provide a plot of glucose values over an extended period of time, such as a month or several months. By highlighting periodic peaks and valleys, these graphs can shed light on whether therapy adjustments are needed for things like menstrual cycles, off/vacation days vs. work/school days, and seasonal variations in physical activity. Trend graphs are also useful for illustrating control changes over prolonged periods of time. Gradual upward trends often indicate a need to intensify therapy. Downward trends may indicate that your therapy is on the right track as long as you are not experiencing hypoglycemia too often. In Figure 4-4 below, the trend graph shows that glucose levels are becoming steadily less erratic and more consistent.

Figure 4-4. Example of a glucose trend graph

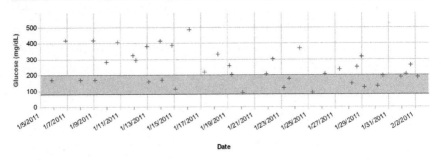

Carbohydrate Gram Counting

As mentioned in the previous chapter, carbohydrates are the primary blood sugar–raising elements in the diet. All carbohydrates (simple and complex), with the exception of fiber, convert into blood glucose fairly rapidly. Thus, quantifying the carbohydrates in our meals and snacks is of the utmost importance.

For those who are attempting to match their mealtime rapid-acting insulin to food intake, carbohydrates should always be counted in *grams*. This is the most precise and practical way to count carbs; using carb "choices" or "exchanges" tends to make things more complex and less precise. If you are accustomed to using the exchange or choice system, the transition to grams can be made by using Table 4-4 below. Simply add the amount of carbohydrates you are getting from each exchange, and you have your carb total for your meal.

Table 4-4. Converting exchanges into grams of carbohydrate

1 bread exchange	= 15 grams carb
1 fruit exchange	= 15 grams carb
1 milk exchange	= 12 grams carb
1 vegetable exchange	= 5 grams carb
1 meat exchange	= 0 grams carb
1 fat exchange	= 0 grams carb

In other words, a meal consisting of two breads, two fruits, a milk, and three meats contains $(2 \times 15) + (2 \times 15) + (1 \times 12) + (3 \times 0)$, or 72 grams of carbohydrate. Just make sure you have the right portion sizes for each exchange. For example, one ordinary banana may be one, one and a half, or two fruit exchanges, depending on the size of the banana.

As a general rule, counting all carbs equally is best. True, there are some subtle differences in how quickly different carbohydrates raise the blood sugar, but all carbs (except for fiber) eventually turn into glucose, so count them all the same. For example, 12 grams of carbohydrate from milk will raise the blood sugar more slowly than 12 grams of carbohydrate from bread, but after several hours the *total* rise will be equal.

If you consume a food high in fiber, such as whole grain bread, beans, or bran cereal, you may not see as much of a blood sugar rise as you might expect. Fiber is a carbohydrate that is resistant to digestion and hence does not tend to raise the blood sugar. When taking nutrition information from a food label, subtract the fiber grams from the total carbohydrate. For example, a high-fiber cereal that contains 8 grams of fiber and 31 grams of total carbohydrate should be counted as 23 grams of carb (31–8).

Now this is really important: *The more accurate you are at carb counting, the better you will be able to control your blood sugar.* There are a number of techniques for counting carbs. One of the simplest and most effective is label reading. All food manufacturers in the United States (as well as most other industrialized countries) are required to list the serving size, total carbohydrate content, and carbohydrate breakdown on their food labels. Note that food labels include the fiber in the total carbohydrate even though fiber does not convert into blood sugar.

Sugars (simple carbohydrate)
+ Starch/other (complex carbohydrate)
+ *Fiber*
= Total carbohydrate

Figure 4-5. Sample food label

Delicious, Chocolatey

Gloopers

Nutrition Facts	
Serving Size: ½ cup (1 oz)	
Servings Per Container 8	
Amount Per Serving	%Daily Value
Calories 150	
Total Fat 6g	10%
Saturated Fat 5g	25%
Sodium 120 mg	5%
Total Carbohydrate 20g	7%
Sugars 12g	
Protein 2g	3%

Figure 4-5 shows a sample food label: A serving of Gloopers (a half cup) contains 20 grams of total carbohydrate. If you consume a full cup, you would have 40 grams of carb.

Sugar alcohols such as sorbitol, mannitol, and xylitol are also included in the total carbohydrates. Sugar alcohols are used as sweeteners in many sugar-free foods. Although slow to act, sugar alcohols will raise blood sugar, albeit less than most other carbohydrates will. As a rule, it is a good idea to deduct half (50 percent) of the sugar alcohol grams from the total carbohydrate.

Another tool for carbohydrate gram counting is a nutrient guide. There are many pamphlets, books, and websites that list the carbohydrate content of various foods. Some cover specific categories such as restaurant food or ethnic food; others cover a wide range of commonly consumed foods. Several are listed in the resources section in Chapter 10. My book *The Ultimate Guide to Accurate Carb Counting* serves as both a nutrition reference and a detailed teaching guide for becoming a more proficient carb counter. Feel free to visit my website (www.integrated diabetes.com) or call my office (877-735-3648) to order a copy.

A somewhat more sophisticated technique for counting carbs is portion estimation. This method is particularly useful when dining out or enjoying foods that vary in size, such as fresh fruit, starchy vegetables, or baked goods.

Portion estimation involves using a common object such as your fist or a deck of cards to determine the approximate size of a particular food item. Then the carb count is determined based on the typical carb content for a standard size of that item.

Common measuring devices:
    soda can = 1½ cups
    adult's fist = approx. 1 cup
    large handful = approx. 1 cup
    tennis ball = approx. ½ cup
    cupped hand = approx. ½ cup
    child's fist = approx. ½ cup
    tip of thumb = approx. 1 inch across
    adult's spread hand = approx. 8 inches diameter
    adult's palm = approx. 4 inches diameter

Approximate carb counts for standard portion sizes:
    potato ≈ 30g/cup
    pasta (w/sauce) ≈ 35g/cup
    rice (boiled) ≈ 50g/cup
    sticky rice ≈ 75g/cup
    salad/raw vegetables ≈ 5g/cup
    cooked vegetables ≈ 10g/cup
    rolls ≈ 25g/cup
    dense bread (bagel/soft pretzel) ≈ 50g/cup
    fruit ≈ 20g/cup
    ice cream ≈ 35g/cup
    cake/muffin/pie ≈ 45g/cup
    pretzels ≈ 25g/cup
    chips ≈ 15g/cup
    popcorn ≈ 5g/cup
    cereal ≈ 25g/cup
    milk ≈ 12g/cup

juice, soda ≈ 30g/cup
sport drink ≈ 15g/cup
sub sandwich rolls ≈ 8g/inch
pizza ≈ 40g/8-inch diameter (round)
pizza ≈ 30g/closed hand (slice)
cookie ≈ 20g/4-inch diameter
pancake ≈ 15g/4-inch diameter
tortilla ≈ 15g/8-inch diameter

For example, an adult's fist is equal to about a one-cup portion. If a cup of boiled rice contains 50 grams of carbohydrate and you consume one and a half fist-size portions of rice, you will have eaten about 75 grams of carbohydrates. Three large handfuls of chips will contain 3 x 15, or 45 grams of carbohydrates. A six-inch-long sandwich will contain 6 x 8, or 48 grams of carbs.

A more precise technique for counting carbs involves using carb factors. By weighing the portion of food that you plan to eat on a gram scale and multiplying by the food's carb factor, you will obtain a precise carb count. A carb factor is actually the percentage of a food's weight that is carbohydrate. For example, apples have a carb factor of 0.13, which means that 13 percent of an apple's weight is carbohydrate. If an apple weighs 120 grams, the carb content is 120 x 0.13, or 15.6 grams. For an abbreviated list of carb factors, see Appendix B.

When you're ready to put your carb counting skills to the test, try taking the Carb Counting Quiz at my website, http://integrateddiabetes .com/carbquiz.shtml. Solutions and a scoring guide are provided—but no cheating!

Dietary Discipline
Mastering the fine art of carb counting does not give you free reign to consume everything and anything in sight. For one thing, providing the necessary *spacing* between meals and snacks is important. This gives your mealtime insulin a chance to get your blood sugar back down to normal before you eat and thus temporarily drive it up again.

Think of it this way: If you were on a small boat that had sprung a leak, what would you do? If you let the water keep pouring in and just bail out, you're never going to get the water completely out of the boat. But if you seal the leak and then bail, you should have a dry boat in no time. Eating too frequently, without allowing space between meals, is like letting the water continue to pour in—but in this case, it is glucose flowing into your bloodstream. Your blood sugar is never going to come back down to normal because you're constantly adding additional glucose. Waiting a while after eating is like plugging the hole: The mealtime insulin bails the glucose out of your bloodstream and your blood sugar comes back down to normal.

> Spacing meals and snacks at least three hours apart will help you keep your blood sugar levels close to normal.

In my experience it is best to wait at least three hours between meals and snacks. After three hours rapid-acting insulin has done the vast majority of its work so the blood sugar should be close to normal again.

Another aspect of the daily diet that requires attention is the amount of fat intake. As mentioned in Chapter 3, consuming large amounts of dietary fat can cause unusual and unwanted changes to blood glucose levels. Large amounts of fat in a meal can slow digestion to the point that rapid-acting insulin peaks before the blood sugar has a chance to rise. This can produce hypoglycemia soon after eating, followed by a blood sugar rise a few hours later. The fat itself can then cause a secondary blood sugar rise by causing insulin resistance and the liver to oversecrete glucose. Also, don't forget that fat is very high in calories and tends to contribute to unwanted weight gain. This in turn can also cause insulin resistance and increased insulin requirements, and it may further increase your risk for large blood vessel (macrovascular) diseases.

So the bottom line is don't graze, and keep the fat intake modest.

Insulin Dosage Adjustment

By its very nature diabetes management requires ongoing adjustment of insulin doses. Self-adjustment of insulin is necessary to balance the factors that raise and lower blood sugar. Matching insulin to your precise needs is what your pancreas would do if it could. To "think like a pancreas" means to do what your pancreas would have done on its own.

For starters, rapid-acting insulin doses should be adjusted based on

- premeal/presnack blood sugar levels;
- anticipated carbohydrate intake; and
- changes to your usual sensitivity to insulin, which can be caused by
  - physical activity,
  - stress,
  - hormonal changes,
  - illness, and
  - medications.

In addition, adjustments should be made to your overall insulin plan (including basal insulin doses) in the event of recurrent hypoglycemia or hyperglycemia. Insulin dosage adjustment and overall plan changes will be the focal point of the next three chapters of this book.

The Right Attitude

I feel like every week I come across someone who has everything they need to manage their diabetes—the latest high-tech toys, a great plan, and all the self-management education, training, and support in the world. Everything . . . except the attitude needed to make it work. This is a common situation among adolescents, but it can—and does—occur in people of all ages and with varying levels of diabetes experience.

A healthy mental approach to living with diabetes is just as important as the tools and skills outlined above—perhaps even more important. See how you fare in the following areas.

Determination

Exactly where does managing diabetes rank in your set of personal priorities? Although nobody would expect you to place your diabetes self-care above the immediate well-being of your family, it should hold a prominent place in your life—and with good reason. Managing your diabetes enables you to fulfill all your other obligations and enjoy what life has to offer. Think about it: If your diabetes is not in control, how will it affect you at work? At school? At home? At the gym? In bed?

Problem Solving

There will be obstacles to taking care of your diabetes: time constraints, access to care and equipment, other health concerns, and costs. But, as I like to say, when the going gets tough, the tough get *solving*.

For example, if your health insurance is unwilling to pay for a product or service that you feel you need in order to manage your diabetes, fight the company on it. Contact your state's attorney general's office if you suspect that your insurance company is not complying with regulations. And if necessary, pay out of pocket. You simply cannot put a price on your health.

Persistence

Michael Jordan was perhaps the greatest basketball player of all time. A prolific scorer, tenacious defender, and fierce competitor, MJ managed to win six NBA championships despite being undersized—he was a mere six-foot-six—and lacking a dominant "big man" in his supporting cast. But did you know that Michael "Air" Jordan, icon of the basketball world, was cut from his high school basketball team as a freshman? Had Michael chosen to throw in the towel and concentrate on baseball or—heaven forbid—his studies, he would have deprived himself and the rest of the world of his amazing talents.

Persistence is a valuable trait in many aspects of life. From business to dating to basketball, persistence has a way of paying off in big ways. This is certainly the case when managing diabetes. Given the relentless nature of this disease, managing over the long term takes tremendous persistence.

Over the course of your life with diabetes, there will be countless setbacks. When they occur, do not give up. It really helps to live your diabetes life one day at a time. You can't change the past, so don't worry about what you did—or didn't do—yesterday. And you certainly can't live tomorrow until tomorrow. Every day represents an opportunity for a fresh start.

Of course, taking temporary breaks from your usual management routine is reasonable—and perhaps necessary—as long as you maintain a level of care that keeps you out of harm's way. For example, take a day or two each month to relax your diet, exercise, frequent monitoring, and record-keeping routine. Just be sure to take your insulin and check your blood sugar at key times of the day.

Discipline

Despite being a general pain in the neck, some *good* things come from having diabetes. We can get seated in restaurants faster. We may be able to get around the long lines at amusement parks. And we also can develop a healthy sense of discipline.

Being disciplined does not mean living like an emotionless robot. Rather, it means sticking to a plan even in the face of distraction and adversity—maybe not all the time, but certainly most of the time. And there is tremendous value to structure and consistency; it eliminates many of the variables that can mess up our control.

Take, for example, avoiding the tendency to snack too often—even after Halloween, when there are little chocolate snacks everywhere. The benefits of spacing meals and snacks several hours apart were described earlier. Also be sure to engage in your usual exercise, even when you just feel like staying in bed. As we discussed in Chapter 3, physical activity can amplify the effects of insulin for up to forty-eight hours, but those who maintain a consistent pattern of exercise usually have more predictable insulin action. Those who exercise off and on usually have a harder time predicting how well their insulin will work.

If you're the weekend warrior type—lots of activity on the weekends, very little during the week—you will probably find that your insulin sensitivity varies considerably. You may be more prone to unexpected lows on Saturday, Sunday, and Monday, when your sensitivity to insulin is very high, and you might see unusual highs on Tuesday, Wednesday, Thursday, and Friday when you lose insulin sensitivity and your insulin fails to work as hard as you expect. By comparison, someone who exercises consistently throughout the week will have a fairly stable level of insulin sensitivity and hence more predictable insulin action.

People who are disciplined about keeping written records, checking blood sugar levels, counting carbohydrates, calculating insulin doses accurately, taking their insulin on time, and seeing health care providers regularly also tend to have more consistent blood sugar control over the long term.

Acceptance

Despite your best efforts, you will not be in perfect control of your diabetes all the time—and that's okay. If a baseball player went to pieces every time he failed to get a hit, we would have a lot of .300 hitters sitting in the dugout crying.

Set your expectations at a realistic level. Using the "acceptable range" chart earlier in this chapter might serve as a good starting point. If you are in-range 20 percent of the time currently, see if you can get it up to 30 or 40 percent by next month. And remember that even those with outstanding control are still out of range on a semiregular basis.

As Clint Eastwood's Dirty Harry character liked to say, "A man's gotta know his limitations." Accept that there are limits to what you can reasonably accomplish; trying to change too many behaviors all at once usually leads to disappointment and burnout. Making a list of all the things you could be doing to improve your control and then prioritizing them may help. Try to implement one at a time.

For example, if you are just getting started with trying to manage your diabetes intensively, try implementing one key change each week:

Week 1: Start checking your blood sugar before each meal and snack, and then write down the results. Don't worry about what the numbers are—just check and record.

Week 2: Start using a formula to adjust your mealtime insulin doses based on your premeal/presnack blood sugar.

Week 3: Begin looking up the carb counts in your foods and writing them down, along with your blood sugars and insulin doses.

Week 4: Learn to adjust your insulin doses based on carbohydrate intake.

Week 5: Start getting some daily exercise, and add that to your written records.

Week 6: Learn to adjust your insulin doses based on physical activity.

Week 7: Try downloading your meter and evaluating the reports to see if adjustments to your dosing formulas are needed.

Week 8: Send a batch of thank-you brownies to the author of your favorite diabetes book. (My address, incidentally, is 333 E. Lancaster Ave., Ste. 204, Wynnewood, PA 19096. Please don't forget the rest of my staff . . . our office manager is especially fond of brownies!)

Keep in mind that your diabetes records—including blood sugar levels—are simply pieces of information that you and your health care team can use to make competent decisions and fine-tune your management plan. These records are not meant to pass judgment on you as a person. As I tell many of my patients: "Any information is good information—regardless of the numbers." When you look at your logs and downloaded reports, pretend you're the health care provider evaluating someone else's data. Don't take anything too personally!

Finally, memorize the Serenity Prayer. Don't misunderstand: I am not a very religious person, but I do know when something makes sense. The Serenity Prayer reminds us that not everything is within our control. To fret over things beyond your control is a waste of time and effort. Instead, concentrate on the things you can control. We may not have the final say over what each blood sugar reading is, but we can improve our odds of a decent reading by doing the right things.

A little bit of luck—or help from above—wouldn't hurt either.

THE SERENITY PRAYER

*God, grant me the serenity to accept the things
    I cannot change,
the courage to change the things I can,
and the wisdom to know the difference.*

Chapter Highlights

- The HbA1c is an important test for assessing overall glycemic control.
- Establish target glucose ranges based on your personal goals, and strive to hit the targets as often as possible.
- Successful diabetes management requires proper tools, self-care skills, and the right attitude. One or two out of three won't cut it—all three are necessary.
- Self-management tools include appropriate insulin, an effective insulin-delivery device, a modern blood glucose monitoring system, and a supportive, multidisciplinary health care team.
- Self-management skills include appropriate self-monitoring, the ability to organize and analyze your own data, accurate carb counting, dietary discipline, and the capacity to self-adjust insulin doses.
- Attitude traits that contribute to success in diabetes self-care include determination, persistence, discipline, acceptance, and the ability to problem solve.

5

The Basal/Bolus Approach

So you've got all your key components in place. Your home is littered with used test strips. Your carb-counting skills rival those of the diabetes gods. You're even keeping written records for the first time in your life. Now all you need is the right insulin program to make it all pay off.

If you're going to think like a pancreas, your insulin program should include the two Bs: "basal" or "background" insulin, along with "boluses" or "bunches" of insulin at mealtimes.

Basal Insulin

The liver is a fascinating organ. It does about a hundred different things, but one of its main functions is to store glucose (in a dense, compact form called "glycogen") and secrete it steadily into the bloodstream in order to provide your body's vital organs and tissues with a constant source of fuel. This is what keeps your heart beating, brain thinking, lungs breathing, and digestive system, uh, digesting pretty much all the time.

In order to transfer the liver's steady supply of glucose into the body's cells, the pancreas normally secretes a small amount of insulin into the bloodstream every couple minutes. This is called basal insulin. Not only does basal insulin ensure a steady energy source for the body's cells, but it also keeps the liver from dumping out too much glucose all at once. Too little basal insulin—or a complete lack of insulin—would result in a sharp rise in blood sugar levels.

So you might say that basal insulin and the liver are in equilibrium with each other. The basal insulin should match the liver's secretion of glucose throughout the day and night. In the absence of food, exercise, and rapid-acting/mealtime insulin, the basal insulin should hold the blood sugar level nice and steady.

Each person's basal insulin requirement is unique. Typically, basal insulin needs are highest during the night and early morning, and they are lowest in the middle of the day. This is due to the production of blood sugar–raising hormones during the night as well as enhanced sensitivity to insulin that comes with daytime physical activity. Figure 5-1 below illustrates how various hormones play a role in the liver's glucose output. Two hormones in particular—cortisol and growth hormone—cause the liver's natural ebb and flow in glucose secretion.

Figure 5-1. The influence of hormones on the liver's glucose secretion

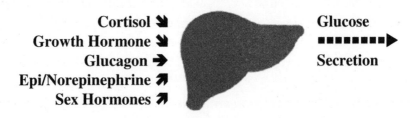

Figure 5-2 shows typical basal insulin requirements for people with insulin-dependent diabetes. The chart is based on data from several hundred insulin pump users whose basal insulin levels were carefully adjusted and fine-tuned.

Although no significant differences were found in the basal insulin requirements for men and women, age does play a significant role. During a person's growth years (prior to age twenty-one) basal insulin

Figure 5-2. Typical basal insulin levels by age group

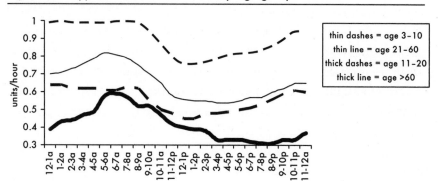

needs tend to be relatively high throughout the night, drop through the morning hours, and gradually increase from noon to midnight. Most adults (age twenty-one-plus) exhibit an abrupt increase in basal insulin requirements during the early morning hours, followed by a drop-off until noontime, a low/flat level in the afternoon, and a gradual increase in the evening. This peak in basal insulin during the early morning hours is commonly referred to as a dawn phenomenon.

The pattern of basal insulin requirements reflects the amount and timing of cortisol and growth hormone secretion within each age category. The youngest group (younger than ten) requires approximately 40 percent less basal insulin than those eleven to twenty, but the twenty-four-hour pattern of peaks and valleys is remarkably similar. Likewise, the oldest group (over sixty) requires approximately 33 percent less basal insulin than those in the twenty-one to sixty age group, but they have a similar twenty-four-hour pattern.

> Basal insulin patterns are dictated mainly by when the body produces hormones that influence the liver's secretion of glucose.

Basal insulin can be supplied in a variety of ways. Intermediate-acting insulin (NPH) taken once daily will usually provide background insulin around the clock, albeit at much higher levels four to eight hours after injection and at much lower levels after sixteen to twenty-four hours. Long-acting basal insulins (glargine and detemir) offer relatively peak-less insulin levels for approximately twenty-four hours. Insulin pumps deliver rapid-acting insulin in small pulses throughout the day and night. With a pump the basal insulin level can be adjusted and fine-tuned to match your body's ebb and flow in basal insulin needs. Combining various forms of long-acting insulin to simulate the body's normal basal insulin secretion is also possible.

The following figures illustrate the action profiles of various types of basal insulin programs.

Figure 5-3. Basal insulin supplied by NPH at bedtime

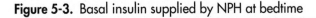

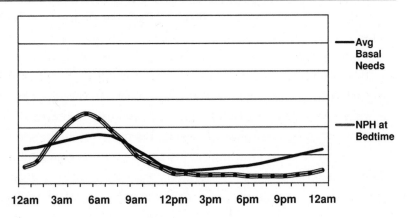

The main advantage of this program is the peak that occurs during the predawn hours. The disadvantages include the unpredictability of the peak (due to NPH's varied rate of absorption from day to day), the potential for low glucose in the early morning (due to the significant peak during the night), and the likelihood that late afternoon/evening blood sugar will rise as the NPH tapers off.

The advantages of this program are the peak in basal insulin during the night and the possibility of using the morning NPH peak to cover the carbs eaten at lunchtime. The drawbacks are the same as those in Figure 5-3 above, plus the major issue of having to conform to a rigid meal/snack schedule during the day due to the peak of the morning NPH insulin. As the graphic clearly shows, this type of basal insulin

Figure 5-4. Basal insulin supplied by NPH in the morning and evening

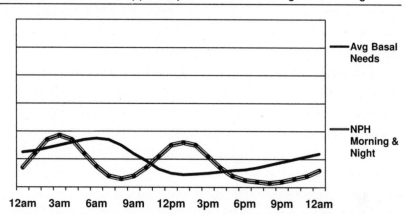

program does a poor job of matching the body's needs. It rarely produces stable glucose levels, particularly during the daytime.

Unfortunately, those who use premixed insulin twice daily are, essentially, utilizing this approach for their basal program. Each injection of premixed insulin contains anywhere from 50 to 75 percent NPH insulin, with the remainder being either regular or rapid-acting insulin.

Glargine (Lantus) is usually taken once daily, but sometimes it is taken twice, particularly when low doses are being used. Detemir (Levemir) is usually taken twice daily, but occasionally it can be taken once a

Figure 5-5. Basal insulin supplied by glargine (Lantus) or detemir (Levemir)

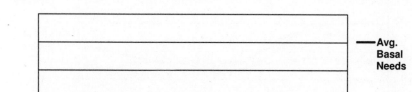

day. When basal insulin is injected twice daily, splitting the doses evenly and taking them approximately twelve hours apart is reasonable. Taking more in the evening and less in the morning does not usually produce a desired peak at any particular time. When taken once daily, it is usually best to take the injection in the morning on a consistent twenty-four-hour cycle. Research has shown that the morning injection has the least potential to cause an undesired blood sugar rise when the insulin is tapering off at around twenty to twenty-four hours.

The main advantage of using glargine or detemir is the relatively unwavering flow of insulin (a very slight peak may occur six to ten hours after injection of detemir) and consistent absorption pattern. The disadvantages include the potential for a gradual blood sugar rise during the night (due to the *lack* of a predawn peak) and around the time of the injection when the insulin is taken once daily, as the basal insulin may wear off a few hours early and take a few hours to kick in. There is also potential for a gradual blood sugar drop in the afternoon as the basal insulin level may exceed the liver's production of glucose.

Figure 5-6. Basal insulin supplied by glargine or detemir plus evening NPH

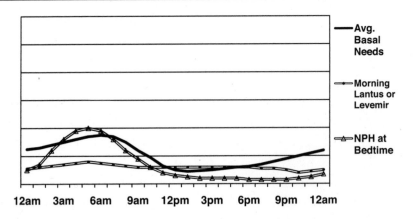

In order to overcome some of the potential problems created by using only basal or NPH insulin to meet the body's basal needs, you can combine the two. When NPH is added at nighttime, glargine or detemir can be taken once daily at a lower dose than if used without

NPH. This minimizes the risk of having glucose levels drop between meals during the day. By adding a modest evening or bedtime dose of NPH, you can achieve a nighttime/early-morning peak. This program offers the unique advantage of allowing day-to-day adjustment of the overnight basal insulin level by making minute changes to the NPH dose without affecting the basal insulin level the following day.

The disadvantages include the need for at least two separate injections and the filling of multiple prescriptions. There is also potential for mixing up doses or taking the wrong insulin at the wrong time because several different types of insulin are being utilized simultaneously.

Figure 5-7. Basal insulin supplied by insulin pump therapy

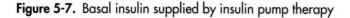
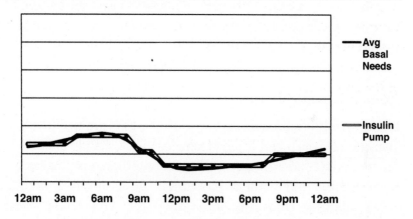

Pump therapy offers the greatest degree of maneuverability in terms of matching basal insulin to the body's needs. Because the pump uses small pulses of rapid-acting insulin to deliver basal insulin, variations in peak or action time are not an issue. Changes can be made to the basal insulin delivery on the hour or half-hour, so you can easily build peaks and valleys into the program. Pumps also permit temporary changes to basal insulin levels in order to accommodate short-term changes in basal insulin needs (for situations such as illness, high/low activity levels, and stress).

Perhaps the greatest drawback to delivering basal insulin with a pump is the risk of ketoacidosis. Any mechanical problem resulting in a lack of basal insulin delivery can result in a severe insulin deficiency in just a few hours. Without any insulin in the bloodstream, the body's cells begin burning large amounts of fat (instead of sugar) for energy. This results in the production of acidic ketone molecules—a natural waste product of fat metabolism. This rarely occurs when taking injections of long-acting insulin because there is almost always some insulin working as long as injections are not missed.

Bolus Insulin

Insulin peaks are necessary because of the rapid blood sugar rise that occurs after eating carbohydrates (sugars and starches). Carbohydrates usually take about ten to twenty minutes to begin raising the blood sugar level, with a high point occurring thirty to ninety minutes following a meal.

Option A: Rapid Insulin

Rapid-acting insulin analogs such as aspart (Novolog/NovoRapid), glulisine (Apidra), and lispro (Humalog) peak sharply about sixty to ninety minutes after injection. You can use these insulins effectively to cover meals and minimize postmeal blood sugar spikes when taken at the right times (usually prior to eating). Rapid insulin is particularly effective when consuming rapid-digesting sugars and starches, such as bread, cereal, potato, rice, pastries, and sugary candies. It also permits the quickest fix for high blood sugar levels.

Option B: Regular Insulin

Regular insulin, by contrast, usually takes thirty minutes to begin working and peaks two to three hours after injection. Due to its relatively slow/inconsistent peak and long duration of action (up to six hours), regular is not usually the preferred insulin to use at mealtimes. Postmeal glucose levels tend to spike up very high for the first couple of hours and then plummet over the next several hours. Taking regular insulin thirty to sixty minutes before a meal mitigates this problem, but this is rarely practical. However, regular insulin can still play a role at mealtimes, particularly when slow-digesting foods are being consumed (we'll discuss this later in the section on postmeal control) or if you have a form of neuropathy called *gastroparesis*, which causes abnormally slow digestion.

Option C: NPH Insulin

In some cases intermediate-acting insulin (NPH) is used to cover a meal or snack that will be consumed four to six hours later. For example, NPH taken at breakfast can be used to cover the carbohydrates eaten at lunch. This may be the only available option for someone who is dependent on a caregiver to administer insulin and the caregiver is not available at lunchtime, such as a young child attending a school with limited nursing resources. However, because of its broad and inconsistent peak, NPH taken in the morning has a tendency to cause the blood sugar to drop before lunch, and it allows for a sharp rise after lunch.

Figure 5-8 below compares how various insulins cover the blood sugar rise that occurs after carbohydrate-containing meals and snacks. As you can see, the insulin analogs (Humalog and Novolog) provide the closest match.

Figure 5-8. Bolus insulin options

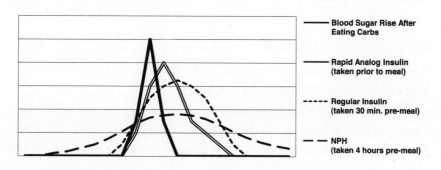

Putting Them Together

Selecting the best insulin program to meet your needs depends on a number of factors. If you have type 2 diabetes, LADA, or are in the honeymoon phase of type 1 diabetes, your pancreas may produce sufficient amounts of insulin to meet either your basal or bolus needs, but usually not both. (A lab test called a *C-peptide* can be performed to see how much insulin your pancreas produces on its own.)

If you still produce some of your own insulin, you can determine your general insulin requirements by doing the following:

- Check your blood sugar level at bedtime, have no snack, and then test first thing in the morning. If your blood sugar rises more than 30 mg/dl (1.7 mmol/l) while you sleep, your pancreas is not making enough insulin to cover your basal needs; you will require supplementary basal insulin. Glargine or detemir are excellent choices because of their steady action and relatively low risk for causing hypoglycemia.
- Check your blood sugar before and again sixty to ninety minutes after eating a meal. If your blood sugar was normal (below 120 mg/dl or 6.8 mmol/l) before eating but rises above 180 mg/dl (10 mmol/l) after eating, you will probably need bolus insulin at mealtimes. In most cases, rapid-acting insulin analogs provide the best mealtime coverage.
- If your blood sugar is usually over 200 mg/dl (11 mmol/l), distinguishing between basal and bolus insulin needs may be difficult. Not to worry: A combination of both should do the trick.

If you have type 1 diabetes or have type 2 and are in need of an aggressive insulin regime, utilizing a program that combines both basal and bolus insulin is best.

To select the basal/bolus insulin program that best meets your needs, the *Consumer Reports* approach can be very helpful. I appreciate the way *Consumer Reports* provides objective, side-by-side comparisons of the various features of competing products. Recognizing that different features are important to different people, this approach makes choosing the products and services that will best meet your individual needs easy.

Here, then, is my "Consumer's Guide" to the most commonly used and recommended basal/bolus insulin programs:

Table 5-1. Gary's non-copyright-infringing comparison of basal/bolus insulin programs

	Overall BG control	Work involved	Hypoglycemia risk	Lifestyle flexibility	$ Price
1. (Pre)mixed twice daily	☹	☺	☹	☹	☺
2. Morning mixed & evening split	☹	☺	☹	☹	☺
3. MDI with bedtime NPH	😐	😐	😐	😐	☺
4. MDI with injected basal	😐	😐	😐	😐	😐
5. MDI with injected basal and bedtime NPH	☺	☹	😐	😐	😐
6. Insulin pump therapy	☺	😐	☺	☺	☹

☺ = good   😐 = fair   ☹ = poor

Option 1: (Pre)mixed twice daily

Prebreakfast: NPH and rapid (in premixed formulation or combined manually)
Predinner: NPH and rapid (in premixed formulation or combined manually)

Figure 5-9. The action profile of NPH and rapid insulin taken twice daily.

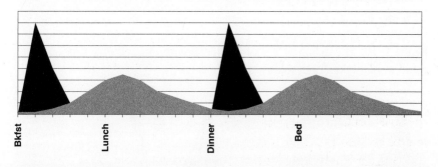

This was a common insulin program back in the 1970s and '80s (with regular insulin instead of a rapid-acting analog). It can be delivered using premixed insulin (70/30 or 75/25) in pen or vial/syringe form, or the user

can combine it in a syringe manually. The premixed formulations have a major shortcoming in that you cannot change the proportion of inter-mediate to rapid insulin. If you need more rapid insulin, you must also take more intermediate (NPH) insulin, and vice versa. With the morn-ing NPH insulin peaking in the afternoon, you must consume meals and snacks at specific times and in specific amounts. Changes to your usual schedule can lead to high and low glucose levels. Exercise during the day can also produce lows with this type of insulin schedule unless you con-sume extra carbohydrates. The evening NPH insulin peaks around mid-night and dissipates as dawn approaches, predisposing most users to low blood sugar in the middle of the night and highs at wake-up.

Perhaps the only advantage to this program is the ease of administra-tion. Only two injections per day are required, and premixed formulations eliminate the possibility of accidentally taking the wrong type of insulin. They also do not require multiple steps to mix the insulins together. Taking NPH insulin twice daily also virtually guarantees that some basal insulin is always present, thus minimizing the risk of ketoacidosis.

Taking two doses of premixed insulin has obvious drawbacks and lim-itations. However, it may prove practical for those who are unwilling or unable to utilize a more sophisticated program safely and consistently.

Option 2: Morning mixed and evening split
Breakfast: NPH and rapid insulin
Dinner: Rapid insulin
Bedtime: NPH

Figure 5-10. The action profile of NPH taken morning and bedtime, and rapid insulin taken at breakfast and dinner

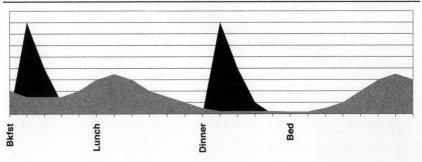

There are a few differences (and improvements) between this program and Option 1. The user mixes the morning dose manually (rather than using premixed insulin), so you can adjust the dose of rapid insulin based on the amount of carbohydrate consumed. Likewise, the dinner rapid insulin is not part of a premixed formulation and can be adjusted as needed. By moving the evening NPH from dinner to bedtime, the peak is shifted to early morning (around the time of the dawn phenomenon), thus improving the chances for stable glucose levels during the night.

Otherwise, the disadvantages still abound. You must structure and monitor midmorning, midday, and afternoon food intake and physical activity carefully. You have little schedule flexibility. And you still have morning and evening injections of NPH that you must take on schedule but whose action profiles may vary from day to day.

This program may be of some practical use for those who depend on a caregiver to administer insulin injections. If the caregiver is unavailable to administer insulin in the middle of the day (e.g., during the school day), you utilize the morning NPH to offset the glucose rise from midday meals and snacks (albeit not very effectively). It may also work for anyone whose schedule is highly consistent from day to day.

Option 3: MDI with bedtime NPH
Breakfast: rapid insulin
Lunch: rapid insulin
Dinner: rapid insulin
Snacks: rapid insulin
Bedtime: NPH

Figure 5-11. The action profile of NPH taken at bedtime and rapid insulin taken at each meal and snack

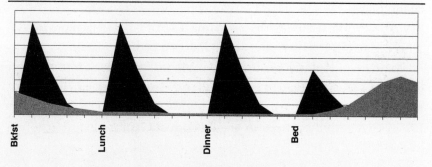

Bkfst   Lunch   Dinner   Bed

Now we enter that zone we call multiple daily injection (MDI) therapy. People used to go to great lengths to avoid taking more injections,
but then reality set in. Rational people came to realize that the injections are probably the *easiest* thing about living with diabetes. The rigid,
restrictive lifestyle and uncontrolled blood sugars are what are really
hard to live with. An MDI program minimizes these types of major
drawbacks, all at the small price of a few extra virtually pain-free injections each day.

With this specific type of MDI program, NPH insulin taken at bedtime provides an early-morning peak to cover the dawn phenomenon
as well as a prolonged "tail" of action that ensures the presence of at
least some basal insulin throughout the day. However, the peak and duration of NPH can vary from day to day, putting the user at risk for
unanticipated high or low blood sugar levels in the morning. Furthermore, the tapering action of the insulin in the afternoon and evening
may result in a blood sugar rise between meals late in the day.

This type of plan requires an injection of rapid-acting insulin at
every meal and snack, although snacks that are very low in carbohydrate may not require an injection. What qualifies as a "free" snack (not
requiring insulin) varies from person to person. In general, the smaller
your body size, the more sensitive you will be to small amounts of carbohydrate. For example, someone who weighs 250 pounds (120 kg) might
be able to tolerate 10 grams of carb without needing any insulin, but
someone who weighs 50 pounds (24 kg) might need insulin for as little
as 3 to 5 grams of carb.

Many people find that insulin pens make frequent injections less of a
chore. Pens that deliver in half-unit or whole-unit increments are available. And for those who despise the needle sticks, an injection port can
be used. (See resource listings in Chapter 10.) Those who use syringes
have the option of mixing their evening dose of NPH with rapid insulin
if needed to cover a high glucose reading or a bedtime snack.

Taking rapid-acting insulin with each meal and snack restores free-
dom of choice because you can match the insulin doses to the amount
of carbohydrate being eaten. It also allows adjustments for variations
in physical activity as well as timely corrections for glucose readings

that are above or below target. Details about fine-tuning mealtime doses of insulin will be covered in Chapter 7.

Option 4: MDI with injected basal insulin

Morning or evening: glargine

—or—Morning and evening: detemir

  and

Breakfast: rapid insulin

Lunch: rapid insulin

Dinner: rapid insulin

Snacks: rapid insulin

Figure 5-12. The action profile of basal insulin taken once or twice daily as well as rapid insulin taken at every meal and snack

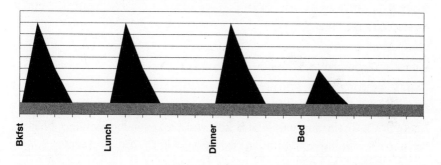

Glargine (Lantus) and detemir (Levemir) are the first insulin formulations that serve as true basal insulins. In some individuals Lantus may show a slight peak six to ten hours after injection and may dissipate earlier than twenty-four hours. But for most people it provides a steady level of basal insulin for about twenty-four hours. Detemir should be taken twice daily due to its shorter duration of action (usually eighteen to twenty-two hours). Each injection of detemir has a mild peak four to ten hours after injection and then tapers off gradually. But when taken twice daily, there are few noticeable peaks and valleys.

Use of basal insulin has its pros and cons. Its consistent absorption and lack of a true peak minimizes the risk of hypoglycemia, although glucose levels may tend to drop gradually between meals during the daytime hours because the dose is usually set high enough to meet basal needs during the night. The peakless nature of these insulins may not be optimal for those with a pronounced dawn phenomenon, whereby basal insulin needs to increase sharply in the early morning hours.

As with any MDI program, injections of rapid-acting insulin are necessary with every meal and snack. And unlike NPH, which can be mixed in the same syringe with rapid-acting insulin, glargine and detemir must be injected separately from rapid insulin.

Option 5: MDI with injected basal and bedtime NPH
Morning: glargine or detemir
    and
Bedtime NPH
    and
Breakfast: rapid insulin
Lunch: rapid insulin
Dinner: rapid insulin
Snacks: rapid insulin

Figure 5-13. The action profile of basal insulin taken in the morning, NPH taken in the evening, and rapid insulin taken at each meal and snack

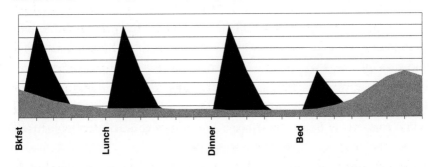

Despite requiring the most injections (two to three shots of basal insulin daily plus rapid-acting insulin at each meal and snack), this program comes about as close as one can get to "thinking like a pancreas" when using injections instead of a pump. A low dose of injected

basal insulin (glargine or detemir) maintains relatively steady glucose levels between meals during the day, and a nighttime dose of NPH offsets the dawn phenomenon in the middle of the night and early morning. The dose of NPH can be adjusted based on factors that might influence overnight glucose levels, such as illness, heavy exercise during the day, and high-fat meals late in the day. For those with a pronounced dawn phenomenon and a need for very flexible dosing of both basal and mealtime (bolus) insulin, this program might be right for you.

Option 6: Insulin pump therapy

Figure 5-14. The action profile of insulin pump therapy

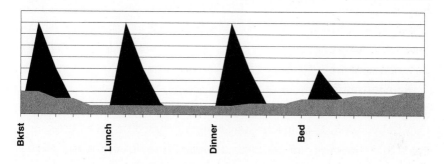

Insulin pumps are beeper-sized, battery-powered devices that infuse rapid-acting insulin just below the skin. Pumps are programmed to deliver tiny pulses of insulin every few minutes throughout the day and night (basal insulin) along with larger doses at mealtimes (bolus insulin). The insulin is delivered by way of a small, flexible plastic tube or a tiny needle called an infusion set. The infusion set must be changed every couple of days in order to prevent clogging and infection as well as to ensure consistent insulin absorption.

The infusion set is usually worn on the abdomen, buttocks, or hip. It adheres securely to the skin and is not likely to pull out while you sleep or exercise. Most feature a disconnect mechanism that allows you to temporarily set the pump and tubing aside for situations such as bathing, contact sports, and intimacy, all while leaving the infusion set portion on/in the skin. The tube that connects the pump to the infusion set is very strong and comes in different lengths. Some pumps stick directly to the skin and don't require any tubing at all. Pumps also have multiple safety features to ensure against accidental insulin delivery.

All pumps are either waterproof or water resistant, and they come with clips that let you attach them to a belt/waistband. A variety of cases, pouches, and fashion accessories make the pump easy to wear in almost any situation. (See Resources in Chapter 10.) A few pumps of-fer remote-control programming so that you don't even have to handle the pump when it comes time to deliver a bolus.

Most of today's pumps have built-in bolus calculators. Enter your blood sugar level and the carbs you plan to eat, and the pump recom-mends a precise dose based on the dosing formulas you and your health care team programmed. Pumps can even deduct previous bolus insulin that is still working in your body so that you don't accidentally overdose yourself. Each pump keeps a record of all this information in its memory for on-screen recall or downloading to a computer.

Some insulin pumps receive data via radio transmissions from blood glucose meters and continuous glucose monitors. This is not to say that they deliver boluses of insulin automatically based on your blood sugar, but rather that they can display the information on-screen and you can then use the information when calculating your boluses.

One very unique aspect of pump therapy is the ability to fine-tune and adjust basal insulin levels throughout the day and night. By match-ing basal insulin to the liver's normal output of glucose, blood sugars should hold steady between meals and during the night. As a result, you can vary your schedule as much as you like in terms of meals, activities, and sleep—in other words, you can live a more normal life. You can also adjust basal insulin levels on the fly for circumstances such as menstrual cycles, pregnancy, stress, illness, travel, high-fat meals, and extended exercise.

One very unique aspect of pump therapy is the ability to fine-tune and adjust basal insulin levels throughout the day and night.

With insulin pumps, you can administer mealtime insulin at the touch of a button—actually, a sequence of button presses. The doses are highly precise; some pumps permit dosing in increments as low as one-fortieth of a unit. All pumps offer the option of delivering mealtime boluses all at once or over an extended period of time—in case you expect your meal to take a while to digest.

Benefits of pump therapy include:

1. **Better blood sugars.** First and foremost, pump users tend to have lower A1cs and less glucose variability (fewer high-to-low and low-to-high swings) than those on injections.
2. **Fewer lows.** By using only rapid-acting insulin, there is no long-acting insulin peaking or working too hard at inappropriate times. This makes pump therapy a good choice for those who have frequent lows, a history of severe lows, or a hard time detecting low blood sugars.
3. **A more flexible lifestyle.** Raise your hand if you can eat, sleep, and exercise at the same times every day. The pump lets you choose your own schedule.
4. **Dose calculations.** Modern pumps come equipped with a bolus calculator that helps you determine mealtime doses based on carb intake, blood glucose levels, and the amount of insulin still active from previous boluses. Imagine that—no math!
5. **Precise dosing.** Pumps deliver insulin to the nearest .1, .05 or .025 units—ideal for those who are sensitive to very small doses, such as children and lean/active adults.
6. **Convenience.** There is no need to draw up syringes every time you need insulin; just reach for your pump and press a few buttons.
7. **No Shots.** Multiple daily insulin injections can be uncomfortable and cause skin problems, but pumps only require a needle stick once every two to three days to change the infusion set.
8. **Easy adjustments for real life.** Temporary basal insulin changes help maintain stable blood sugar during periods of growth, illness, seasonal sports, dining out, and menstruation. The ability

to deliver boluses all at once or over a prolonged period of time can be instrumental in achieving optimal after-meal glucose control.

9. **Weight control.** Eat what and when *you* choose; snacks are not required when you use a pump.
10. **Data analysis.** Insulin pumps store a plethora of historical information that can be displayed on-screen or transmitted to various computer programs for analysis and fine-tuning.

Potential drawbacks to pump therapy include:

1. **Cost.** Although most insurance plans cover insulin pumps and supplies, there are often copays and deductibles that must be met.
2. **A learning curve.** Don't expect good control right away. You usually need a few months to get the basal and bolus doses regulated and adjust to using the pump correctly.
3. **Inconvenience.** Wearing the pump around the clock, even during sleep, can become awkward once in a while. My infusion set tubing gets caught on a doorknob at least once a month!
4. **Technical difficulties.** As mechanical devices, pumps are prone to occasional infusion set clogs, electronic failures, computer glitches, and damage due to typical wear and tear.
5. **Skin problems.** Skin can become irritated from infusion set adhesive, and infections can occur if infusion sets are worn too long or inserted improperly. Insulin absorption can be hindered if you do not change infusion sets regularly and rotate sites properly.
6. **Ketosis.** The absence of long-acting insulin with pump use can present a problem if insulin delivery is interrupted for more than a few hours. Blood sugar can rise very quickly, and ketones may appear in the bloodstream and urine if the problem is not corrected.
7. **Infusion set changes.** Every couple of days you must change your own infusion set. This five- to ten-minute procedure involves nu-

merous steps and can be momentarily uncomfortable or traumatic for the novice pump user.

Certain characteristics and skills are needed to use a pump successfully. After all, just about any idiot with insulin-dependent diabetes and a decent insurance policy can go on an insulin pump, but to succeed with a pump takes preparation and follow-through. The following are some qualities that are most important for those seeking an insulin pump:

- Motivation/interest in going on a pump, keeping in mind that nobody is 100 percent sure that it is right for them until they give it a try. A bit of hesitancy and anxiety about making the switch to a pump are perfectly normal.
- A true state of insulin dependence (type 1 or type 2, with little or no insulin production).
- Adequate resources to afford the pump and ongoing supplies (via insurance or cash).
- Ability to handle basic programming and infusion set change procedures. A guardian can do this if the user is very young or physically/mentally challenged.

Certain skills are essential for making a successful transition to pump therapy. Ideally, these should be mastered prior to starting on the pump:

- carbohydrate counting (using grams rather than exchanges)
- blood glucose monitoring prior to meals and bedtime (four times a day, minimum)
- complete record keeping in paper or electronic form (including blood sugars, insulin doses, carb intake, and physical activities)
- self-adjustment of insulin doses (based on blood sugar levels, carb intake, and physical activity)
- an understanding of the basic principles of pump therapy (including the components of a pump and infusion set as well as the role of basal and bolus insulin)

Successful pump use will also require adequate follow-up and fine-tuning. This should include

- basal rate testing throughout the day and night (fasting for eight- to ten-hour intervals and testing blood sugars to see if they are holding steady);
- fine-tuning of bolus formulas (based on record keeping);
- troubleshooting and preventing emergencies such as DKA (diabetic ketoacidosis); and
- using advanced pump features such as extended boluses and temporary basal rates.

To learn more about pump therapy, contact one of the insulin pump manufacturers listed in Chapter 10 or ask your physician or diabetes educator. Find out if there are insulin pump user groups in your area. Group meetings offer an excellent forum for meeting other pumpers and finding out about their personal experiences since starting pump therapy.

Substitution Is Permitted

When selecting an insulin program, don't think of it as a lifetime commitment. Many people switch plans because of changes in their lifestyle or simply because a particular plan fails to do the job. Several of my clients have tried an MDI program but were unable to achieve the kind of control they wanted, so they made the move to a pump. I have also had pump users who switched back to injections, either permanently or temporarily, due to image concerns or the desire for more structure in their lives. The one constant in life is change—you are not locked into any particular plan.

And what if your physician doesn't agree with your program choice? Ask why. Perhaps they have a good argument that will sway your decision. If not, you might want to look for another doctor. After all, this is your diabetes, and you deserve the right to manage it in the manner that suits you best.

Chapter Highlights

- For an insulin program to be successful, it should include both basal and bolus components.
- Basal insulin may be supplied in the form of NPH, glargine/detemir, or insulin pump therapy. Pump therapy usually provides the best basal insulin coverage.
- Bolus insulin may be supplied in the form of rapid, regular, or NPH insulin. Rapid insulin is by far the most advantageous.
- Various combinations of basal/bolus therapy are possible, each with its own pros and cons. Choose the one that will meet your personal needs the best.

CHAPTER

6

Basal Insulin Dosing

Once you have settled on an insulin program that meets your needs, the next order of business is to determine the right doses. Think of yourself as a giant lump of clay that needs to be molded and sculpted into fine art. (My personal self-sculpture is a cross between Rocky Balboa and Bond, James Bond.) Any artistic creation takes time, so be patient. Make one adjustment at a time, evaluate the results, and then fine-tune before moving on to another area.

Another truism about fine art: Beauty is in the eye of the beholder. What works for some may not work for others. When looking at typical dosing patterns and formulas, use them only as starting points. Individual needs may—no, make that will—vary.

Let's start with the fine-tuning of *basal* insulin levels. Basal insulin serves as the foundation for your entire insulin program. With a solid, level foundation, you can build something great, but with a cracked or crooked foundation, you will need to manipulate everything placed on top of it in order to avoid epic disaster. In diabetes terms, when high or low blood sugars appear, knowing what to adjust is difficult unless you have already established the proper basal insulin levels. That's why it is best to fine-tune your basal doses before attempting to regulate the mealtime/boluses.

In the previous chapter I presented typical basal insulin profiles for people within different age groups. During a person's growth years (prior to age twenty-one), basal insulin requirements tend to be heightened throughout the night. This is due to the production of hormones (primarily growth hormone and cortisol) that stimulate the liver to release extra glucose into the bloodstream. Following one's growth years, the production of these hormones is limited primarily to the predawn hours, causing the liver to secrete extra glucose in the early morning. This is commonly called a "dawn effect" or "dawn phenomenon."

Initial Basal Doses for Those Injecting Insulin

The body's insulin requirements are affected by a number of factors, including body size, activity level, stage of growth, and the amount of endogenous (internal) insulin production from your own pancreas. To find out how much insulin your pancreas is producing, a blood test called a "C-peptide test" can be performed. C-peptide is attached to the insulin molecule when it is first secreted from the pancreas. They call it C-peptide because it is shaped like the letter C (isn't that ingenious!). Enzymes in the blood break this piece off, leaving two parts: the active insulin molecule and the C-peptide. By measuring the amount of C-peptide in the blood, we can determine approximately how much insulin the body is making on its own. A result of less than 0.5 ng/ml indicates that the pancreas is producing abnormally low amounts of insulin.

If you are just getting started with a basal/bolus insulin program, start with a conservative dose and increase gradually until your blood sugar levels are within an acceptable range.

For those with type 2 diabetes who are still producing some of their own insulin, the total daily insulin requirement is often less than 0.5 units per kilogram, or about .2 units per pound, of body weight daily. However, this can vary considerably depending on your body's degree of insulin resistance. For instance, a person with insulin-resistant type 2 diabetes who weighs more than 250 pounds (113 kg) might require hundreds of units of insulin in order to manage blood sugar levels, whereas someone of similar size who still produces some of their own insulin and is only modestly insulin resistant might require only 10 or 20 units of insulin daily.

For individuals who produce virtually no insulin on their own (including those with type 1 diabetes), insulin requirements are somewhat more predictable. Table 6-1 below provides typical ranges for total daily insulin needs.

Table 6-1. Total daily insulin requirements (units per kilogram body weight)

Age ➡ Activity level ⬇	Young children	Adolescents	Adults	Older adults
Mostly inactive	.60–1.2	.80–2.0	.60–1.2	.20–.50
Moderately active	.50–1.0	.75–1.50	.50–1.0	.15–.40
Very active	.40–.80	.60–1.2	.40–.80	.10–.35

For instance, if you are a moderately active adult, you will likely require .50 to 1.0 units of insulin per kilogram of body weight per day. If you weigh 160 pounds, that equals approximately 73 kilograms (lbs x .454 = kg). Your daily insulin need should be in the range of 37 (73 x .50) to 73 (73 x 1.0) units per day.

Given that basal insulin usually accounts for 40 to 50 percent of a person's total daily insulin needs (50 to 60 percent covers food), basal insulin doses typically fall within the ranges shown in Table 6-2 below. Keep in mind that those who eat large quantities of carbohydrate will

Table 6-2. Daily basal insulin requirements (units per kilogram body weight)

Age ➡ Activity level ⬇	Young children	Adolescents	Adults	Older adults
Mostly inactive	.25–.60	.30–1.0	.25–.60	.20–.50
Moderately active	.20–.50	.30–.75	.20–.50	.15–.40
Very active	.15–.40	.25–.60	.15–.40	.10–.35

have a smaller percentage of their daily insulin as basal, whereas those who eat very little carbohydrate will have a larger proportion of basal insulin. Basal insulin needs also tend to drop as we pass from middle to older age.

Translating this to units of insulin, let's look at an example.

Debbie is thirty-eight years old and has type 1 diabetes. She weighs 136 pounds, exercises for an hour every day, and has a very active job.

First, we must convert her weight into kilograms (lbs x .454 = kg).

$$136 \times .454 = 62$$

Because Debbie is a very active adult, she requires .15 to .40 units of basal insulin for every kilogram she weighs.

$$62 \times .15 = 9 \text{ units}$$
$$62 \times .40 = 25 \text{ units}$$

Debbie should require somewhere between 9 and 25 units of basal insulin daily. Because the basal/bolus approach is new to her and she has a history of low blood sugars, she and her physician opt to start conservatively with 10 units of basal insulin.

Let's take another example. Ben is a teenager with type 1 diabetes who gets a moderate amount of exercise and weighs 105 pounds. According to Table 6-2, he will likely require between .30 and .70 units of basal insulin per kilogram of body weight per day.

His weight in kilograms:

$$105 \times .454 = 48$$
$$48 \times .30 = 14$$
$$48 \times .70 = 34$$

Having had mostly high blood sugars recently (as teenagers are prone to do), Ben and his physician elect to start somewhere in the middle, with 25 units of basal insulin.

One more example: Jackie is sixty-eight years old and has type 2 diabetes that is poorly controlled on oral medications. Her doctor has determined that her pancreas makes very little insulin. She weighs 210 pounds and gets hardly any exercise.

Her weight in kilograms:

$$210 \times .454 = 95$$

According to Table 6–2, she will likely require between .20 and .50 units of basal insulin per kilogram of body weight.

$$95 \times .20 = 19$$
$$95 \times .50 = 48$$

Given that Jackie is fairly insulin resistant, she and her physician choose to start with a dose of 40 units of basal insulin.

Fine-Tuning Injected Basal Doses

When injecting basal insulin, our goal is to find a dose that maintains steady blood sugar levels through the night (or while sleeping, for those who work night shifts). Ideally, the doses of glargine, detemir, or nighttime NPH should produce no more than a 30 mg/dl (1.7 mmol/l) change while sleeping—assuming that before you go to sleep you do not eat, take rapid-acting insulin, or perform heavy exercise.

> The right dose of basal insulin should keep the blood sugar fairly steady through the night.

A consistent rise or drop of more than 30 mg/dl (1.7 mmol/l) indicates a need to change the basal insulin dosage. To determine whether your overnight basal insulin dose is set correctly, follow this procedure:

1. Have a fairly healthy dinner (not too much fat; avoid restaurant and take-out food). High-fat food will cause a prolonged blood sugar rise and will alter the test results. Take your usual doses of dinnertime rapid-acting insulin and long-acting/basal insulin.
2. If you normally exercise in the evening, go ahead and do so, but keep the intensity and duration modest. Very heavy exercise may cause the blood sugar to drop several hours later, which would also influence the test results.
3. At least three hours after dinner, perform a bedtime blood sugar check. As long as your blood sugar level is above 80 mg/dl (4.4 mmol/l) and below 250 (13.9 mmol/l), do not take any food or rapid-acting insulin and proceed with the experiment. If you are below 80 (4.4), take a snack and try the test another night. If you are above 250 (13.9), give a correction dose of rapid-acting insulin and try again another night. If you repeatedly have high or low readings at bedtime that keep you from beginning the test, consider making an adjustment to your dinnertime food, insulin, or medication.
4. Check your blood sugar again in the middle of the night (or the middle of your sleep time) and first thing in the morning (upon waking up). You need the middle-of-the-night reading to rule out a potential Somogyi Phenomenon (see page 133).

If your blood sugar rises or falls less than 30 mg/dl (1.7 mmol/l) from bedtime to wake-up time, congratulations! Your basal insulin dose looks good. If it rises more than 30 mg/dl (1.7 mmol/l), increase your basal insulin dose by 10 percent and repeat the test. If it is dropping by more than 30 mg/dl (1.7 mmol/l), decrease your basal insulin by 10 percent and repeat the test. Continue adjusting and repeating the test until your blood sugar holds reasonably steady through the night.

For example, let's say you're taking 10 units of detemir in the morning and 10 at night. If your bedtime blood sugar reading was 185 mg/dl (9.2 mmol/l) and your wake-up reading was 122 mg/dl (6.8 mmol/l), your basal insulin dose is too high, as the blood sugar dropped by 63 mg/dl (2.4 mmol/l) while you slept. Had your bedtime blood sugar been closer to normal, you probably would have experienced hypoglycemia during the night. Reduce the detemir to 9 units both morning and night, and run the test again the following night.

Had the blood sugar risen from 87 mg/dl (4.8 mmol/l) to 160 mg/dl (8.9 mmol/l)—a rise of 73 (4.1)—an increase in the basal insulin would be in order.

If your bedtime reading was 95 mg/dl (5.3 mmol/l) and you woke up at 77 mg/dl (4.3 mmol/l), shout woo-hoo! You would not need to adjust the basal insulin dose because the blood sugar changed by only 18 mg/dl, or 1 mmol/l, during the night.

Attack of the Killer Somogyi

What about that pain-in-the-neck reading you took in the middle of the night? No one likes having their sleep interrupted (unless, of course, your hot partner is looking for some action). So that extra reading had better be worth it. Believe me, it is.

In many instances, a blood sugar drop during the night—particularly to levels below 70 mg/dl (3.9 mmol/l)—causes the body to secrete hormones that raise the blood sugar by morning, all without your knowledge. This occurrence, known in the medical community as the "Somogyi Phenomenon" (named after its discoverer), can interfere with basal dosing decisions if it goes undetected.

Consider the following example, illustrated in Figure 6-1. Larry and his two brothers, Daryl and Darryl, all have diabetes (now *there's* a gene pool to avoid). They each take glargine for their basal insulin. Each starts and finishes the night with the same blood sugar increase. Without knowing the blood sugar in the middle of the night, our first instinct would be to increase the basal insulin for all three. But a closer look at the data in Table 6-3 reveals more effective solutions.

Larry is experiencing a sharp blood sugar rise soon after he goes to sleep. This could be considered an early "dawn phenomenon." Adding a small dose of NPH at dinnertime or a small dose of rapid insulin at

Figure 6-1. Three routes to high blood sugar in the morning

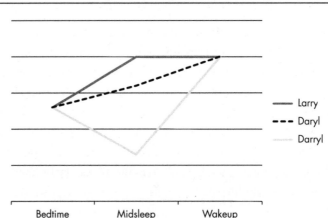

Bedtime   Midsleep   Wakeup

- Larry
- - - Daryl
- Darryl

Table 6-3.

	Bedtime	Midsleep	Wakeup
Larry	130 mg/dl	190 mg/dl	200 mg/dl
	(7.2 mmol/l)	(11.1 mmol/l)	(11.1 mmol/l)
Larry's brother **Daryl**	130 mg/dl	160 mg/dl	200 mg/dl
	(7.2 mmol/l)	(8.9 mmol/l)	(11.1 mmol/l)
Larry's other brother **Darryl**	130 mg/dl	65 mg/dl	200 mg/dl
	(7.2 mmol/l)	(3.6 mmol/l)	(11.1 mmol/l)

bedtime would probably resolve this problem. An insulin pump might also be a good option for Larry because he could program it to deliver a little more basal insulin during the early part of the night.

Daryl experiences a steady rise through the night, so an increase in his glargine dose should do the trick.

Darryl, however, is experiencing a Somogyi Phenomenon. He is dropping to mildly low levels in the middle of the night and rebounding to a higher level by morning. Increasing his basal insulin would make the problem worse, not better. But a reduction in his basal dose, or possibly adding a bedtime snack, would make the most sense.

Initial Basal Doses for Insulin Pump Users

Basal insulin delivered by an insulin pump comes in the form of tiny pulses of rapid-acting insulin infused every few minutes throughout the day and night. Rapid-acting insulin tends to work more efficiently than longer-acting insulin, so there is less waste. As a result, the average pump user requires approximately 20 percent less basal insulin than those who take intermediate- or long-acting insulin by injection.

I prefer to start pump users on one flat rate of basal insulin and then fine-tune using the methodology described later in this chapter. Of course, one flat rate is not likely to meet your needs adequately. But to make assumptions about when and how much of a basal peak you need based on your injection program could be a big mistake. There may be major differences in your basal insulin pattern when transitioning to pump therapy, so it is best to start conservatively in order to avoid unexpected lows.

To determine an initial rate of basal insulin delivery, two approaches are available: the formula methods (which provide a very rough approximation) and the empirical approach (which provides a less rough approximation).

One of the formula methods is based on your current insulin injection program:

1. Add up all the units of insulin you take in an average day, including basal and bolus insulin.
2. Divide the total in half (assuming that 50 percent of your insulin is going to be basal and the other half bolus).
3. Multiply by .8 (to take away 20 percent of the total dose, because basal delivered in the form of rapid-acting insulin tends to work more efficiently than basal delivered as long-acting insulin).
4. Divide by 24 (to figure the hourly rate).

For example, Marley took three injections daily (before going on the pump):

Breakfast: 18 NPH and 5 units Novolog (on average)
Dinner: 8 units Novolog (on average)
Bedtime: 12 units NPH

Marley's total insulin for the day is 43 units.
　　Half that amount is 21.5 units.
　　Taking away 20 percent leaves 17.2 units.
　　Dividing by twenty-four hours, we get .7 units per hour.

Another formula calculation is based on body weight. Anyone going directly onto the pump without ever having taken insulin injections should use this method.

1. Take your weight in pounds. To convert kilograms to pounds, multiply by 2.2.
2. Divide by 10 (a magic number . . . trust me on this).
3. Divide by 24 (to figure the hourly rate).

If Ben weighs 195 pounds (88.5 kg), we divide 195 by 10 to get 19.5, and divide this by 24 to get .8 units per hour.

A more effective method for determining starting basal insulin doses on the pump involves taking your current insulin program, breaking it down into basal and bolus components, and then taking the basal total to figure your hourly rate. Once you determine the injected basal insulin, I recommend you still take away 20 percent when figuring the initial basal requirements on the pump.

Using Marley's insulin program as an example (see above), I would figure that none of her Novolog doses are used as basal insulin. Because she does not take any insulin at lunchtime, I would assume that approximately 50 percent of her morning NPH serves as basal insulin (the remainder covering lunch and daytime snacks), and 75 percent of her nighttime NPH serves as basal insulin (the remainder covering some of her night snack and some of breakfast). Thus, 50 percent of 18 (9 units) plus 75 percent of 12 (9 units) are being used as basal insulin, for a total of 18. I would then take 20 percent away to come up with

14.4 and then divide by 24 to come up with an initial rate of .6 units per hour.

For someone taking a long-acting basal insulin, I would simply take 20 percent away from the total daily dose of glargine or detemir and divide by 24 to come up with an hourly basal rate.

For example, if Karen is on the following program:

Breakfast: 8 units lispro (on average), 12 units detemir
Lunch: 6 units lispro (on average)
Afternoon snack: 3 units lispro (on average)
Dinner: 8 units lispro (on average)
Bedtime: 2 units lispro (on average), 13 units detemir

I would ignore the lispro doses completely and figure that the detemir is the only basal insulin. Taking 20 percent away from her 25 total units of detemir, we come up with 20 units. Dividing by 24 hours, we get a starting rate of 0.8 units per hour.

Fine-Tuning Pump Basal Rates

When you go on an insulin pump, whatever you do, *don't just assume that the initial basal settings are correct.* This is one of the biggest mistakes you can make. The power of the insulin pump is its ability to deliver varied amounts of basal insulin at different times of day.

The purpose of basal insulin is to match the amount of glucose the liver secretes into the bloodstream. The right basal rate is one that keeps your blood sugar at a fairly constant/steady level when you have not eaten or bolused for several hours and are not exercising. You must establish appropriate basal rates in order to obtain quality blood sugar control and enjoy the flexible lifestyle the pump affords.

Testing, adjusting, and retesting basal rates can be a bothersome process, but it is well worth the effort. To determine whether your basal insulin rates are set properly, you will need to wait approximately four hours after your last bolus and meal/snack and then observe what happens. This will give the carbs time to finish digesting and the bolus time to finish working. The conditions that must be met in order to run a successful basal test are listed below.

No food should be digesting.

- Wait at least four hours after your last meal/snack before beginning the test.
- The meal/snack preceding the basal test should be low in fat. (No restaurant food or take-out; these tend to raise blood sugar for many hours).
- Do not consume any calories during the basal test unless your blood sugar drops below 80 (4.4). Even fat and protein can affect blood sugar levels. You may have water or diet beverages during the test.
- Avoid caffeinated beverages during the basal test. (Caffeine can cause blood sugar to rise.)
- Do not consume alcohol in the meal/snack preceding the basal test. (Alcohol can reduce the liver's normal glucose secretion.)

No bolus insulin should be working during the basal test.

- Wait at least four hours after your last bolus to begin the test (six hours if using regular insulin).
- The bolus given for the last meal/snack should be delivered normally (not extended in any way).
- Do not bolus during the test unless your blood sugar rises above 250 (13.9).

Your body should be producing its normal amount of glucose.

- Do not perform the test if you have had a low blood sugar within the previous four hours. (Hypoglycemic episodes tend to produce a hormonal response that can raise the blood sugar for several hours.)
- Do not run the test if you are ill or experiencing unusual stress.

- Do not run the test if you are taking a steroid medication unless it is a medication that you plan to continue taking indefinitely at a steady dose.
- Avoid testing just prior to or at the start of your menstrual cycle.

Allow basal insulin to be delivered at its normal rate.

- Do not put the pump into suspend just before or during the test.
- Do not disconnect from the pump just before or during the test.
- Do not run a temporary basal rate just before or during the test.
- Do not change your infusion set just before or during the test.

Maintain your normal level of physical activity.

- Do not exercise during the blood sugar evaluation phase of your basal test.
- You may perform light/moderate exercise soon after your pretest meal/snack if you normally do so at that time.
- Perform your usual daily activities during the basal test.

I usually start by testing and fine-tuning the nighttime basal rates. Once you have matched the overnight rate to your liver's output of glucose, your blood sugar should hold steady through the night. This will make testing the morning segment easier, followed by the afternoon segment and, finally, the evening segment.

To start the test, follow these steps:

1. Check your blood sugar at the start of the chosen time period. Remember, you should wait at least four hours since the last bolus of rapid-acting insulin.
2. If the blood sugar is above 250 (13.9), bolus for the high blood sugar and cancel the test. If below 80 (4.4), eat to bring your blood sugar up and cancel the test. If the blood sugar is not too high or too low, proceed with the test.

3. During a basal test, check your blood sugar with a fingerstick reading every couple hours. Less frequent testing may cause you to miss a temporary rise or fall. Alternatively, collect your data using a continuous glucose monitor.

Basal testing should be set up around the framework of your usual mealtimes and sleep patterns. The schedule shown below in Table 6-4 can be used as a general guide for performing a complete set of basal tests. Running the basal tests for longer periods of time is fine if you can tolerate fasting for more than eight to ten hours at a time, as is breaking the daytime tests into smaller intervals (e.g., for young children).

Table 6-4. Example basal testing schedule

Test	Eat and bolus no later than	Check blood sugar at	Okay to eat and bolus again after
Overnight	7 p.m. (eat dinner, then skip evening snacks)	1 p.m., 1 a.m., 3a.m., 5 a.m., 7 a.m.	7 a.m.
Morning	3 a.m. (have a bedtime snack, then skip breakfast)	7 a.m., 9 a.m., 11 a.m., 12 p.m.	12 p.m.
Afternoon	8 a.m. (have breakfast, then skip lunch and afternoon snacks)	2 p.m., 2 p.m., 4 p.m., 6 p.m.	6 p.m.
Evening	2 p.m. (have a late lunch, then skip afternoon snacks and have a late dinner)	6 p.m., 8 p.m., 10 p.m., 11 p.m.	11 p.m.

If pricking your finger mercilessly doesn't appeal to you, another excellent way to collect basal testing data is by wearing a continuous glucose monitor. Say what you will about CGMs: They are not always as accurate as we would like them to be, but when they show an upward trend, you can bet your family jewels that your blood sugar is rising. And when they show a downward trend, you are almost certainly dropping. So because basal testing is all about checking the stability of blood sugar levels in a fasting state, a CGM can serve as an ideal source of information, not to mention that it saves you from waking up during the night to prick your finger!

Grounds for Adjustment

Whether you use fingerstick or CGM data, if your blood sugar drops more than 30 mg/dl (1.7 mmol/l) during the test period, the basal rate is probably too high. If it rises more than 30 mg/dl (1.7 mmol/l), the rate is most likely too low. You should adjust and retest the basal rate (the next day, if possible) to determine whether the adjustment is working. Continue to adjust and retest until you obtain a reasonably steady result.

If the result of a basal test appears to be very erratic (rises, falls, rises, falls), try repeating it the next day to see if a similar pattern appears. Inconsistent readings usually mean that an unforeseen variable is affecting the results. Likewise, if the glucose level rises or falls by a huge amount, the cause may be something other than the basal insulin being a bit off. Again, repeat the test to see if the results are similar.

Quantity of Adjustment

The amount of the change made to basal rates depends on a number of factors, including your sensitivity to insulin, the magnitude of the blood sugar change during the basal test, and the precision of your pump. For someone on relatively large doses of insulin, making tiny, infinitesimal basal adjustments is like trying to take down a charging rhino with a water pistol. Likewise, making relatively large changes if you are on very small doses is like shooting a mosquito with a bazooka—there might be a bit of collateral damage. Hopefully you get the idea. Table 6-5 should serve as a useful starting point.

Table 6-5. Suggested magnitude of basal insulin adjustments

		Current basal level (units/hr)		
		0.0–0.35	.4–1.0	>1.0
Blood sugar change during Test	Modest (30–60 mg/dl; 1.7–3.4 mmol/l)	.025 or .05	.10	.20
	Large (>60 mg/dl; >3.4 mmol/l)	.05 or .10	.20	.30

Timing of Adjustment

Having diabetes teaches us that we need to plan ahead. Increasing (or decreasing) a basal rate at 6 p.m. is not going to affect the blood glucose *at 6 p.m.* Basal rates need to be changed one to two hours *prior* to observed blood sugar changes because the rapid-acting insulin the pump infuses does the majority of its work one to two hours after delivery. I prefer to make changes two hours ahead for most adults and one hour ahead for most children and very lean/active adults.

For example, if an adult's blood sugar rises between 3 a.m. and 7 a.m., I would recommend increasing the basal rate between 1 a.m. and 5 a.m. If a child's blood sugar drops between 8 p.m. and 1 a.m., I would recommend a basal reduction between 7 p.m. and 12 a.m.

Incidentally, even though most pumps allow basal rates to be adjusted on the half-hour, I prefer to make setting changes on the hour (i.e., 1:00 rather than 1:30). Remember, basal insulin is made up of tiny boluses of rapid-acting insulin, and rapid insulin works over a three- to four-hour period. Basal insulin levels in the body don't change dramatically all at once; there is more of a gradual shift. Thus I simply find it more practical and manageable to make changes on the hour.

Quality of Adjustment

When setting up a twenty-four-hour basal program, our objective is to mimic normal physiology as closely as possible. A healthy pancreas secretes basal insulin in a circadian pattern, based mainly on how other hormone levels vary during the course of a full day. It produces more basal insulin at certain hours, less at others. Normally, there is one peak period and one valley period—not multiple peaks and valleys. A basal program that includes multiple peaks and valleys is almost always incorrect—or at least compensating for some other aspect of the insulin program that is not set up properly. For example, consider the basal pattern in Figure 6-2.

Figure 6-2. Basal pattern with one peak and one valley

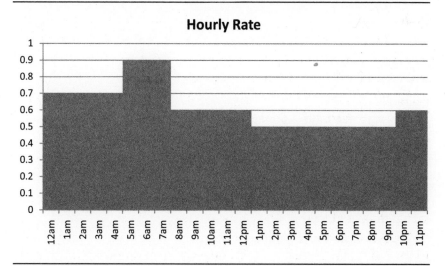

12 a.m.–5 a.m.: .70
5 a.m.–8 a.m.: .90
8 a.m.–1 p.m.: .60
1 p.m.–10 p.m.: .50
10 p.m.–12 a.m.: .60

This pattern has one peak (between 5 and 8 a.m.) and one valley (1 to 10 p.m.). It has integrity, as far as basal programs go.

Now consider the pattern in Figure 6-3.

Figure 6-3. Basal pattern with multiple peaks and valleys

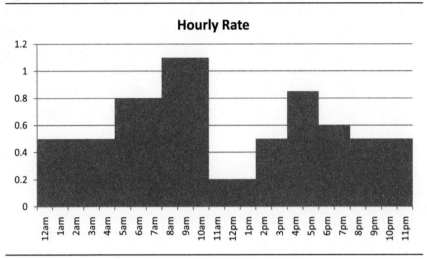

Hourly Rate

12 a.m.–5 a.m.: .50
5 a.m.–8 a.m.: .80
8 a.m.–11 a.m.: 1.10
11 a.m.–1 p.m.: .20
1 p.m.–4 p.m.: .50
4 p.m.–6 p.m.: .85
6 p.m.–8 p.m.: .60
8 p.m.–12 a.m.: .40

This program has two peaks: a big peak from 7 to 10 a.m. and a smaller peak from 4 to 6 p.m. Given that the basal rate is .5 continuously from 2 p.m. until 7 a.m. *except* for those few hours in the late afternoon, the 4 to 6 p.m. rates may be set inappropriately. Perhaps the basal peak in the late afternoon is compensating for an afternoon snack that is not covered sufficiently with a bolus.

Examples

The following are examples of basal tests and the recommended adjustments for each.

April is a compulsive forty-one-year-old accountant who recently started using a pump and has a flat basal rate of 1.2 units per hour throughout the day and night. To verify her overnight basal rate, she had a low-fat dinner at 6 p.m. and nothing else to eat the rest of the night. Her blood sugars through the night were as follows:

10 p.m.: 117 mg/dl (6.5 mmol/l)
12 a.m.: 187 (10.4)
2 a.m.: 238 (13.2)
4 a.m.: 240 (13.3)
6 a.m.: 218 (12.1)

April's blood sugar rose sharply between 10 p.m. and 2 a.m. and then held steady from 2 a.m. until 6 a.m. (the slight drop-off from 4 to 6 a.m. is likely due to the loss of some sugar through the urine). Based on this, I would recommend that she increase her basal rate by .3 units per hour (to 1.5) from 8 p.m. until 12 a.m. and repeat the early phase of the test (taking readings just until 2 a.m.). Her basal rate from 12 a.m. until 4 a.m. appears to be set correctly, as the blood sugar level remained fairly constant from 2 a.m. to 6 a.m.

Mindy is a manipulative ten-year-old whose basal rates are .20 units per hour from 3 a.m. until 9 a.m., and 0.15 units per hour the rest of the day. To confirm her morning basal rate, her parents had her skip breakfast and check her blood sugars through the morning (they promised her a Happy Meal for lunch if she complied). The results were as follows:

7 a.m.: 184 mg/dl (10.2 mmol/l)
8 a.m.: 192 (10.7)
9 a.m.: 177 (9.8)
10 a.m.: 190 (10.6)
11 a.m.: 224 (12.4)
12 p.m.: 259 (14.4)

Mindy's blood sugar held steady from 7 a.m. to 10 a.m., so the .2 basal from 6 a.m. to 9 a.m. looks good. The blood sugar rise from 10 a.m. to 12 p.m. requires a basal increase to 0.20 from 9 a.m. to 11 a.m. Mindy's parents could combine her next (afternoon) test with a recheck of late morning by having her eat breakfast at 6 a.m. and then perform blood sugar checks from 10 a.m. until 2 or 3 p.m.

Lily is an artsy-fartsy college student using an insulin pump. Her current basal rates are as follows:

12 a.m.–7 a.m.: 0.5 units/hr
7 a.m.–1 p.m.: 0.4 units/hr
1 p.m.–8 p.m.: 0.3 units/hr
8 p.m.–12 a.m.: 0.4 units/hr

Lily noticed that her blood sugars in the morning were higher than they were at bedtime, so she decided to wear a continuous glucose monitor for a week. She was careful not to snack after 8 p.m. so that we could find out what was going on. The results are shown below in Figure 6-4:

Figure 6-4

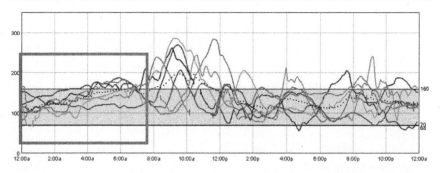

As you can see in the box, her glucose levels were rising steadily through the night from approximately 1 a.m. to 6 a.m. She was not dropping low and then rebounding to a higher reading (Somogyi Phenomenon), and because she was not eating after 8 p.m., food was probably not causing the rise. So Lily concluded that she needed to increase her basal insulin by .1 from midnight through 5 a.m.

Paul has been using a pump for a short while and also uses a continuous glucose monitor. His current basal rate is flat at .8 units per hour. He found that he was experiencing frequent lows since starting on the pump, but he wasn't sure if the problem was too much basal or too much bolus insulin. Here is a look at a day's CGM data for Paul.

Figure 6-5

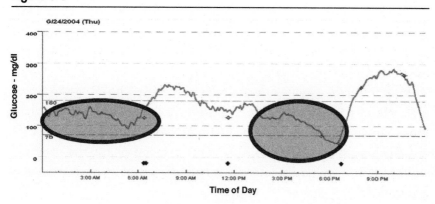

Notice in the ovals that his blood sugar is dropping starting after 3 a.m. and after 3 p.m., both approximately four hours after his last bolus was given. This indicates that his basal insulin dose is likely too high. Paul reduced his basal rate from .8 to .7 units per hour and began a series of scheduled basal tests to fine-tune his overall program.

Idiosyncrasies about Basal Testing

Life is never simple when you have diabetes. Basal insulin levels and basal testing don't always follow the rules according to Hoyle. There are a few "quirks" that you should be aware of.

For starters, never test your basal rates the first day or night when you start on your pump or injected basal insulin program. You need at least twenty-four hours (and sometimes as long as forty-eight hours) for previously injected long-acting insulin to clear from your body.

Anytime the blood glucose level is above 180 mg/dl (10 mmol/l), the kidneys will channel some sugar into the urine. This may produce a slight decrease in the blood sugar concentration. Thus, when performing a basal test with elevated blood sugars, a slight drop-off in the blood sugar is to be expected and does not necessarily mean that the basal setting is too high.

In some people even near-lows will cause a hormonal response that induces a mild blood sugar rise. Again, this does not necessarily mean that the basal setting is too low.

After finishing a fasting test, don't be surprised to see a significant spike in the blood sugar soon after eating. This is a natural response to fasting; the digestive system puts food on the fast track to reaching the bloodstream.

In terms of the basal patterns observed, people who are still producing some of their own insulin tend to have flatter basal profiles than those who are truly insulin-dependent. For those with type 2 diabetes or LADA as well as type 1s still in a honeymoon phase, the pancreas will adjust its own insulin secretion to offset some of the peaks and valleys in the liver's glucose secretion.

Beyond Basal Basics

In addition to allowing the user to set a multitude of different basal delivery rates throughout the day and night, all pumps can store settings for more than one complete twenty-four-hour program. Alternate basal programs can be useful during periods of heightened insulin need (such as sick days, travel days, or prior to menstruation) or decreased insulin need (such as days filled with physical activity or postmenstruation). Use of alternate basal programs will be discussed in more detail in Chapter 8, along with the use of short-term basal rate adjustments called "temporary basal rates."

Obviously, fine-tuning basal insulin levels can become complex. This is a great opportunity to work with members of your health care team who specialize in this sort of thing—most likely your CDE or pump trainer. And if you don't have local access to someone who really knows their stuff, give my office a call! We consult people worldwide via phone and the Internet, so you're never without options. We even offer a class at Type-1 University (www.type1university.com) that focuses specifically on the ins and outs of fine-tuning basal insulin.

Remember, *you* are the ultimate decision maker regarding your diabetes plan, but it never hurts to seek out expert advice!

Chapter Highlights

- Basal insulin is the foundation of your entire insulin program.
- Basal insulin's job is to match the liver's output of glucose. It should hold your blood sugar steady in the absence of food, exercise, and bolus insulin.
- Basal insulin usually makes up 40 to 50 percent of the total insulin for the day.
- For those taking basal insulin by injection, the right dose should keep your blood sugar from changing more than 30 mg/dl (1.7 mmol/l) through the night.
- Pump users should test and fine-tune their basal settings at each phase of the day and night.
- Basal programs typically feature one peak and one valley.

CHAPTER

7

Bolus Calculations

Ahhh, pizza, hot from the oven. The aroma of freshly popped popcorn. Cold Italian ice on a warm summer day. That mysteriously tasty cream center in Oreo cookies.

Basal insulin would meet our needs just fine . . . if we never ate. But we do eat (praise the lord!), and the carbohydrates in the things we eat make blood sugars rise. So for everything from Philly pretzels to Philly cheesesteaks as well as countless other culinary delights, we have something called bolus insulin.

> Boluses are bunches of rapid-acting insulin used to cover carbs or lower high blood sugar levels.

Boluses are bunches of rapid-acting insulin given to cover the blood sugar rise that the carbohydrates in our meals and snacks produce. Boluses are also used to lower blood sugars that are higher than we want. Boluses can be adjusted based on several factors, including the amount of rapid insulin that is currently working and our level of physical activity before and after eating. There are many other secondary factors that influence bolus requirements; these will be discussed in the next

151

chapter. For our purposes here, we will focus on the four primary factors that are used to determine bolus doses:

1. the amount of carbohydrate in the meal or snack
2. the blood sugar level at the time of the meal or snack
3. the amount of insulin still remaining from previous boluses
4. the amount of planned (or completed) physical activity

For those of you who are mathematically inclined (you know who you are—your checkbooks actually balance each month), boluses are calculated as follows:

The bolus dose = (food dose + correction dose – insulin on-board) x activity adjustment

Later in this chapter we will also discuss the importance of bolus *timing* in order to keep the blood sugar from rising too high or dropping too low after eating.

For now, let's focus on what makes up the ultimate bolus dose of insulin.

Part 1. Insulin to Cover Carbs

As is the case with basal insulin, appropriate bolus insulin dosing requires individualization and fine-tuning. Each person's needs are unique. To match insulin to food, we use something called an "insulin-to-carb (I:C) ratio." In other words, we need to determine how many grams of carbohydrate each unit of rapid-acting insulin covers. For example, a 1-to-10 (1:10) ratio means that one unit of insulin covers 10 grams of carbohydrate, and a ratio of 1-to-20 (1:20) means that each unit covers 20 grams. If you have basic math skills (or a calculator or an electronic dosing guide—see resources section), figuring the food bolus is easy. Simply divide your carbs by your ratio. If each unit covers 10 grams and you consume 65, you will need 6.5 units of insulin (65 divided by 10 = 6.5).

> An insulin-to-carb ratio tells us how many grams of car-
> bohydrate each unit of insulin covers.

I:C ratios may seem a bit backward at first. A ratio of 1:10 will produce a larger insulin dose than a ratio of 1:15. A snack containing 30
grams of carb will require 3 units if you're using a 1:10 ratio, but only
2 units if you're using 1:15. As the second number in the ratio goes up,
the amount of insulin goes down.

The beauty of an I:C ratio is that it gives you the flexibility to eat as
much or as little carbohydrate as you choose while still maintaining control of your blood sugars. However, *spacing meals and snacks at least a few
hours apart (three or more hours is optimal) remains important* so that bolus
insulin can return the blood sugar to normal before you eat and raise it
again. Even if carbs are counted—and bolused for—carefully, controlling blood sugar when grazing is almost impossible. Frequent munching
puts you in a perpetual state of an after-eating blood sugar rise, waiting
for the bolus to kick in and bring things back down to normal.

Incidentally, requiring different I:C ratios at different times of day is
common. This is due to changes in hormone levels and physical activity, which affect insulin sensitivity. Many people find that they need
their lowest I:C ratio—and thus their highest bolus—at breakfast and
their highest ratio—and lowest bolus—in the middle of the day. For
example, I personally need 1u:10g carb at breakfast, 1u:16g carb at
lunch, and 1u:14g at dinner.

If you already take rapid-acting insulin at your meals and your blood
sugar levels are close to normal most of the time, figuring your I:C ratio
is easy. Simply add up the grams of carb in your usual meals and divide
by the units of rapid-acting insulin.

For instance, Sam usually devours 45 grams of carb at breakfast and
takes 5 units of rapid acting insulin. His blood sugar before breakfast
and before lunch are similar, so it appears that each unit of insulin covers 9 grams of carb (45 divided by 5).

If you have never used an I:C ratio for calculating your mealtime insulin, don't worry: There are a number of ways to set up an initial ratio. Whichever method you choose, starting with a conservative dose is best (are you getting tired of hearing that yet?). It is better to run your blood sugar a little high than too low because frequent lows are dangerous and will make evaluating and fine-tuning your dosing formulas very difficult.

The 500 Rule

The 500 rule is based on an assumption that the average person consumes (via meals and snacks) and produces (via the liver) approximately 500 grams of carbohydrate daily. By dividing 500 by the average number of units of insulin you take daily (basal plus bolus, also called "total daily dose" or TDD), you should get a reasonable approximation of your I:C ratio: *500/TDD*.

For example, if you take a total of 25 units of insulin in a typical day, each unit of insulin should cover approximately 20 grams of carbohydrate (500/25 = 20). If you take 60 units daily, your I:C ratio would be 1:8 (500/60 ≅ 8). (See Table 7-1.)

Table 7-1. Determining I:C ratio from total daily insulin

Total daily dose of Insulin (basal + bolus)	Approx. I:C Ratio
8–11	1:50
12–14	1:40
15–18	1:30
19–21	1:25
22–27	1:20
28–35	1:15
36–45	1:12
46–55	1:10
56–65	1:8
66–80	1:7
81–120	1:5
>120	1:4

The advantage to this approach is its simplicity: Only one nice round number to divide (or one easy chart to look at). The obvious weakness to this approach is that it assumes that all people are equally sensitive to insulin and eat about the same amount of food. When using this approach, those who eat very little will tend to receive too little mealtime insulin, and those who eat a great deal will tend to receive too much. This approach also assumes that the amount of insulin you are taking now is appropriate for you. If your blood sugar is frequently above or below your target range, the I:C ratio derived from this approach will likely be incorrect.

The Weight Method

This approach is based on the fact that insulin sensitivity diminishes as body mass increases; each unit of insulin will cover less food in a heavier person than in a lighter person. To determine a starting I:C ratio, divide 1,800 by your weight in pounds, or 850 by your weight in kilograms:

$$1800/\text{wt (lbs)} \qquad\qquad 850/\text{wt (kg)}$$

Table 7-2. Determining I:C ratio from weight

Weight (lbs)	Weight (kg)	Approx. I:C Ratio
<60	<27	1:30
60–80	27–36	1:25
81–100	37–45	1:20
101–120	46–54	1:17
121–140	55–64	1:14
141–170	65–77	1:12
171–200	78–91	1:10
201–230	92–104	1:8
231–270	105–123	1:7
>270	>123	1:5

One of the potential problems with the weight method is that it fails to consider body composition. An individual who weighs 250 pounds but is very muscular will be much more sensitive to insulin than a person of similar weight who has a great deal of body fat. Another problem is that this system fails to consider stages of growth and hormone production. A growing adolescent will require significantly more mealtime insulin than an older person who weighs the same amount. Likewise, a woman who is pregnant will require considerably more insulin than a person of similar weight who is not pregnant. (Insulin patterns during pregnancy will be discussed in detail in Chapter 8.)

Fine-Tuning and Verifying I:C Ratios

You should establish proper basal insulin levels before you attempt to fine-tune your boluses. Any basal insulin changes made after fine-tuning your boluses will require additional bolus adjustments.

Fine-tuning I:C ratios is best done empirically (what my people call "trial and adjustment"). And be sure to assess the I:C ratio at each meal and snack separately because insulin sensitivity changes throughout the day.

Detailed written records are helpful in verifying and fine-tuning I:C ratios. You should also eliminate factors other than food that might be affecting your blood sugar levels. For example, do not include data collected during or after strenuous exercise unless you do so every day at the same time. Also, don't look at information collected during an illness or major emotional stress, at the start of a menstrual cycle, or after a low blood sugar. You should not include meals with very high fat content or unknown carb content (such as heavy restaurant meals) in your analysis.

To analyze your data, take a look at your blood sugar level before the meal and then again at least three hours later (to give the insulin a chance to finish working), without taking in calories or bolus insulin in between. Because strange things can happen on any given day, I like to consider one to two weeks of data when coming to a decision regarding the I:C ratio.

For example, consider the data in Table 7-3:

As you can see, the conclusions sometimes contradict each other (remember, this is diabetes—nothing is ever simple!). However, we can

Table 7-3. Example log sheet

Date	Prebreakfast blood sugar in mg/dl (mmol/l)	Carbs (grams)	Bolus insulin (units)	Prelunch blood sugar in mg/dl	Conclusion
6/1	175 (9.7)	50	6.5	101 (5.6)	1:8 makes BG drop
6/2	83 (4.6)	50	4.0	78 (4.3)	1:12 held BG steady
6/3	62 (3.4)	75	5.0	226 (12.5)	Don't count—low to start
6/4	151 (8.4)	50	6.0	93 (5.2)	1:8 makes BG drop
6/5	210 (11.6)	40	6.0	113 (6.3)	1:7 makes BG drop a lot
6/6	75 (4.2)	75	5.0	180 (10.0)	1:15 makes BG rise
6/7	123 (6.8)	50	5.0	86 (4.7)	1:10 makes BG drop a bit
6/8	99 (5.5)	90	7.0	52 (2.8)	1:14 makes BG drop ???
6/9	97 (5.4)	30	2.5	114 (6.3)	1:12 held BG steady
6/10	154 (8.5)	65	3.0	274 (15.2)	1:20 makes BG rise a lot

still come to a general conclusion based on the results. I would be tempted to assign an I:C ratio of 1 unit per 12 grams of carb. Here's why:

First, I would throw out the data on June 3 due to the low reading prior to breakfast (it most likely led to a rebound high). I would also throw out the data on June 8 because it is inconsistent with every other result, and the meal was much larger than usual (perhaps it was a slow-digesting Denny's Grand Slam breakfast). The rest of the data indicates that an I:C ratio higher than 1:12 produces a blood sugar rise; less than 1:12 produces a drop. When used, 1:12 held the blood sugar fairly steadily, as the lunch readings were within 30 mg/dl of the breakfast readings.

Another technique for evaluating I:C ratios is to analyze the data from a continuous glucose monitor. CGM downloading offers the unique opportunity to see distinct patterns following meals. With a quick look at a single chart, we can determine whether mealtime insulin doses are too high, too low, or on target.

For example, take a look at Figure 7-1. On most days the dinner bolus produces hypoglycemia two to three hours later. If the current

I:C ratio at dinner is 1u:15g carb, trying a lower dose, such as 1u:20g carb, makes sense.

Figure 7-1. Modal day chart from Dexcom CGM

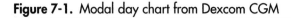

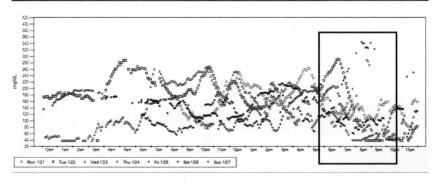

By contrast, the data in Figure 7-2 indicates that the blood sugar is rising and staying elevated after dinner. If the current dinner formula is 1u:15g, increasing the dose to, say, 1u:12g carb to see if this produces better results would be worthwhile.

Figure 7-2. Glucose modal day report from Freestyle Navigator CGM

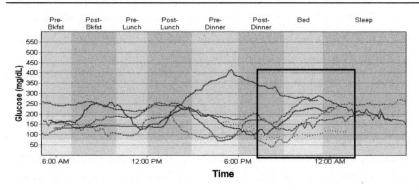

Figure 7-3 reveals the after-meal blood sugar patterns for several days. Apparently, the blood sugar is usually above target (the shaded rectangular areas represent the postmeal target) three to four hours after the mealtime insulin was given. The statistics below the graphs indicate above-target postmeal averages. Based on this information, this person should probably increase the I:C ratio at each meal.

Figure 7-3. Sensor overlay by meal chart from Medtronic CGM

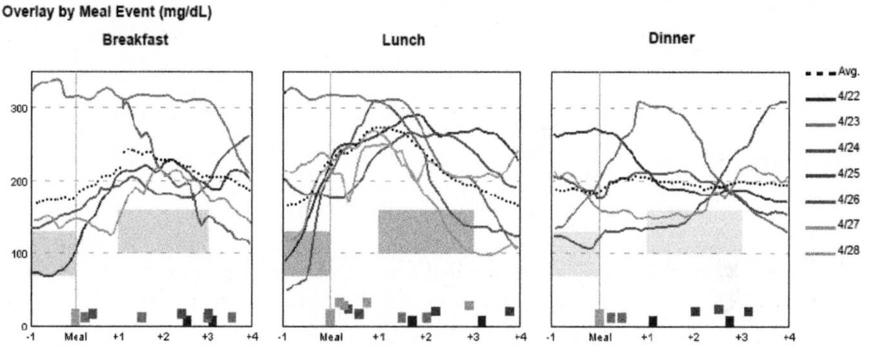

Overlay by Meal Event (mg/dL)

	Sleeping 3:00 AM - 6:00 AM	Before Breakfast	After Breakfast	Before Lunch	After Lunch	Before Dinner	After Dinner	Evening 11:00 PM - 3:00 AM	All Time Periods
Range	100 - 150	70 - 130	100 - 160	70 - 130	100 - 160	70 - 130	100 - 160	100 - 150	
Average SG	146	173	227	190	234	186	195	162	185
High SG	248	340	318	326	312	270	302	308	340
Low SG	56	68	138	48	100	106	134	72	48
Standard Dev.	50	95	51	76	50	51	42	59	65
# of Readings	180	48	119	72	144	60	120	252	995

When analyzing your blood sugar records, the more details, the better. You might discover subtle factors that influence your blood sugar levels and require insulin dose adjustments.

For example, one of my clients, Betty, had blood sugar readings that were above target every Sunday at lunchtime, but normal readings the rest of the week. The reason? Church. Betty is very passionate about Sunday morning services. In addition to sitting still for several hours, the adrenaline rush she gets from prayer was producing a blood sugar rise. The solution: Use her usual 1:10 formula at breakfast during the week, but increase to 1:8 on Sundays.

Another patient, David, was experiencing very inconsistent blood sugars prior to dinner despite having the same lunch each day and using a 1:15 bolus formula every day at lunchtime. In reviewing his records, we found that most of his dinnertime lows were preceded by morning workouts; most of his dinnertime highs were on nonexercise days. The solution: Use a 1:10 formula at lunch after sedentary mornings, but decrease to 1:20 following morning exercise.

Fine-tuning I:C ratios can be a challenging proposition, even for highly trained and experienced health professionals. Given the complexities of determining I:C ratios, having a second set of eyes look over your records is worthwhile. Don't hesitate to ask your physician or diabetes educator to review your data just to confirm that your conclusions seem reasonable. Or give my office a call; my team would be happy to work with you on the fine-tuning process.

(Food Dose + Correction Dose – Insulin On-Board)
x Activity Adjustment

Part 2. Insulin to Correct Blood Sugar

Okay, you've counted your carbs and applied your I:C ratio to determine the food dose. What's next?

The second component of the bolus calculation is the "correction dose": the adjustment to the standard meal bolus to fix blood sugars that are either above or below target. This adjustment improves your chances of having a blood sugar reading that is within your target range before the next meal.

To fully understand this concept, imagine a world-famous archer (green tights and all) named Sir Gary of Kinwood. Sir Gary is trying to win the beautiful Maid Debbie's hand by winning an archery contest. As Sir Gary focuses on his goal (the target, not Maid Debbie), what should he aim for? The bull's-eye, of course! If he aims toward the sides or edges of the target, his chances of hitting the bull's-eye are greatly reduced. In fact, he might miss the target completely, resulting in a chorus of laughter from the evil sheriff's luxury suite.

Remember, blood sugar control is far from an exact science; we're happy just to hit the target *somewhere*. To do so, we must always aim for the center. If your target range is 60 mg/dl (3.3 mmol/l) to 140 mg/dl (7.8 mmol/l), aim for 100 (5.5). If your range is 70 (3.8) to 170 (9.4), aim for 120 (6.7). If your acceptable range is 80 (4.4) to 200 (11.1), aim for 140 (7.8). By aiming for the center, you increase your chances of landing within your target range.

> Your target blood sugar should be a single number near the midpoint of your acceptable target range.

Here's how correction boluses work. If you designate your target blood sugar as 120 mg/dl (6.7 mmol/l) and your premeal reading happens to be 175 (9.7), you will need to add extra correction insulin to your meal dose. Does this guarantee that you will be on target at your next reading? No, but it sure increases the odds that your blood sugar will come down somewhat and land within your target range. If you don't add any correction insulin, it's like aiming to be 175 (9.7) again next time. In archery terms, it's like aiming for the outer edge of the target instead of the bull's-eye.

Sometimes correction boluses involve taking insulin *away* from your usual meal dose. If your blood sugar is 80 (4.4) and your target is 110 (6.1), you will need to deduct some insulin from your meal dose. This increases your chances of raising the blood sugar somewhat and being within the target range by the next meal. If you don't reduce your meal dose when your blood sugar is below your target, you increase your chances of missing the target completely and experiencing a low blood sugar before the next meal. Incidentally, if your blood sugar is below target and you don't plan to eat, there is nothing to deduct the correction dose from. A small snack should take you up toward your target blood sugar.

To figure out the correction dose of insulin, three pieces of information are needed:

1. Your current blood sugar level.
2. Your target blood sugar.
3. Your *sensitivity* factor (sometimes called a "correction factor"). This has nothing to do with how good a listener you are or your willingness to miss a football game for the sake of going shopping

with your partner. Rather, your sensitivity factor is how much each unit of insulin is expected to lower your blood sugar.

Each person's sensitivity to insulin is unique. In general, the heavier you are and the more insulin you take, the less sensitive you will be to each unit. Certain conditions (growth, pregnancy, premenses, illness, stress, surgery, use of steroid medications) also reduce insulin sensitivity, albeit on a temporary basis.

Determining your sensitivity factor is similar to determining your I:C ratio. We start with an estimate based on a mathematical formula and then fine-tune based on actual blood sugar results.

The formula that I find works best for figuring the *daytime* correction factor is called the 1700 (94) rule. Take your total daily insulin, including basal and bolus insulin, and divide into 1700 (94 if measuring blood sugar in mmol/l).

When choosing an initial sensitivity factor, I recommend leaning toward the higher end of the range. For instance, if you average 80 units a day, you might choose 25 (1.4) as your initial sensitivity factor. This reduces the risk of overcorrecting your highs and winding up with low blood sugar. Below are some examples.

Stan takes an average of 28 units of insulin daily. Applying the 1700 rule, we get:

$$1700 / 28 = 61 \ (94 / 28 = 3.4)$$

This means that every unit of rapid-acting insulin should lower his blood sugar approximately 61 mg/dl, or 3.4 mmol/l. To simplify the calculation and start off conservatively, we'll round up to 65 (3.5).

Because Stan's target blood sugar is 110 (6.1), he should add 1 full unit for every 65 (3.5) points over 110 (6.1) . . . and subtract 1 unit for every 65 (3.5) points below 110 (6.1). Expressed as a formula, his correction dose is:

In mg/dl: (current blood sugar − 110) / 65
In mmol/l: (current blood sugar − 6.1) / 3.5

Table 7-4. Estimating the sensitivity factor based on total daily insulin

Average total daily insulin (units) (all basal + all boluses)	Approx. Sensitivity factor (mg/dl) how much 1 unit lowers blood sugar	Approx. Sensitivity factor (mmol/l) how much 1 unit lowers blood sugar
5	320–360	18–20
7	220–260	12–14
10	155–185	8.6–10.3
12	125–155	6.9–8.6
15	95–125	5.3–6.9
18	80–110	4.4–6.1
20	70–100	3.9–5.5
25	60–80	3.3–4.4
30	50–70	2.8–3.9
35	40–60	2.2–3.3
40	35–50	2.0–2.8
45	30–45	1.7–2.5
50	30–40	1.7–2.2
60	25–35	1.4–2.0
70	20–30	1.1–1.7
80	20–25	1.1–1.4
100	15–20	0.8–1.1
120	13–17	0.7–1.0
140	11–15	0.6–0.8
160	10–12	0.5–0.7
180	9–11	0.5–0.6
200	8–10	0.4–0.6

If Stan's blood sugar is 210, we get (210 − 110) / 65, or 1.5 units. He needs 1.5 extra units to correct his blood sugar down to 110. If he needs 3 units for his meal and has a premeal blood sugar of 210, he would increase the dose to 4.5.

If Stan's blood sugar is 76, we get (76 – 110) / 65, or –0.5 units. He needs to take away .5 unit from his meal dose. If he needs 3 units to cover the carbs in his meal and has a blood sugar of 76, he should decrease the dose to 2.5.

Let's look at another example. Nalani takes a total of 75 units of insulin daily. Each unit should lower her blood sugar 23 mg/dl (1700 / 75 = 23), so we'll round up to 25.

If Nalani's target blood sugar is 120, she will add 1 full unit for every 25 points over 120 and subtract 1 unit for every 25 points below 120. Her correction formula is:

$$\text{(current blood sugar} - 120) / 25$$

If Nalani's blood sugar is 171, she will need (171 – 120) / 25, or 2 units, in addition to the insulin she gives to cover her food. If her blood sugar is 310, she will need (310 – 120) / 25, or approximately 8 extra units.

Sensitivity Factors May Vary

You may have noticed the word *daytime* used above when describing the sensitivity factor derived from the 1700 rule. That's because sensitivity to correction boluses can vary based on the time of day, just like I:C ratios often vary from meal to meal. In particular, don't be surprised if each unit of insulin lowers your blood sugar more at night and the early morning than it does during the rest of the day. In the evening many people experience a drop-off in hormones that counteract insulin. As a result, each unit of insulin can lower the blood sugar more at bedtime and in the middle of the night. From my experience, sensitivity factors tend to run 30 to 50 percent higher at night than during the day.

So if you're just getting started using correction boluses and have determined that your daytime sensitivity factor is 40 mg/dl (2.2 mmol/l), you might consider increasing it to 60 (3.3) at night—at least until you have a chance to try it out a few times to see how it works.

Sensitivity factors may also change over time. With weight gain, most people lose some sensitivity to insulin, so the sensitivity factor tends to decrease. Changes in physical activity levels can also affect insulin sensitivity. Prolonged periods of inactivity due to illness, injury, travel, or sedentary occupations may lower insulin sensitivity and require a reduction in the sensitivity factor. Likewise, long-term increases in physical activity can produce the opposite effect.

Verifying Your Sensitivity Factor

You can verify the accuracy of your sensitivity factor by doing the following:

1. Test your blood sugar at least four hours after your most recent bolus of rapid-acting insulin.
2. If the blood sugar is elevated, calculate and give the appropriate dose of insulin. Go about your usual activities, but do not eat or exercise for the next several hours.
3. Test your blood sugar four hours later.
4. Calculate how much your blood sugar came down and then divide by the number of units you gave. This should come close to your sensitivity factor. If it does not, repeat the process the next day. If the results are similar to those from the first day, adjust your sensitivity factor accordingly.

For instance, yesterday I checked my blood sugar four hours after lunch, and it was 205 mg/dl (11 mmol/l) (darned undercounted hoagie!). Applying my daytime formula of (BS – 100) / 40, I gave 2.6 units using my insulin pump. Several hours later, just before dinner, my blood sugar was down to 112. I dropped 93 points (205 – 112). Dividing by 2.6 units, I come up with a sensitivity factor of 36 points per unit—not exactly 40, but close enough!

CGM can also be used to verify whether your sensitivity factors are set correctly. In Figure 7-4, a nighttime correction bolus for high blood sugar brought the level down below target. This indicates that the sensitivity factor may be set too low, which means that each unit drops the blood sugar more than anticipated.

Figure 7-4. CGM demonstrating the results of a nighttime correction bolus

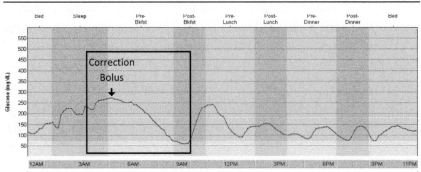

(**Food Dose + Correction Dose** - Insulin On-Board)
x Activity Adjustment

Part 3. Bolus Insulin On-Board

Patience is a virtue. Unfortunately, we all know people who refuse to abide by that philosophy. They want everything right away—no time to putz around with something that isn't working: Fix it, change it, replace it *now*.

Sometimes, things have a way of working themselves out—if given a chance. Take, for instance, insulin. The fastest insulin on the pharmacy shelves still takes about four hours to complete its job. Four hours. Not ten minutes. Not one hour. Not even two hours. Blood sugar measurements taken within a few hours of a bolus will usually still be elevated because the bolus has not yet finished working. So what is one to do? Blast away at the elevated blood sugar with a fully loaded correction bolus? Or sit there helplessly, hoping and waiting for it to come down?

For those of us who want to manage our blood sugar aggressively but prefer not to be thrust into hypoglycemic seizures, the best option lies somewhere in the middle. And this is all about accounting for the insulin that is still working from previous boluses.

This still-working insulin actually goes by many different names, depending on who you're talking to: IOB (Insulin On-Board), BOB (Bolus On-Board), Active Insulin, Insulin Remaining, and so forth. For those of you unfamiliar with the concept of IOB (let's just call it IOB because that saves me a few keystrokes), it refers to the amount of bolus insulin that was previously delivered but is still active (working) in your body. This is important to know because it prevents "stacking" insulin when bolusing for high blood sugars within a few hours of a previous bolus.

For instance, I—like many of you, I'm sure—don't like the feeling of being in the 200s. I used to check my blood sugar a few hours after eating, and if it was elevated, I would apply my usual correction bolus formula. And sure as sugar, I'd wind up low a few hours later.

Nowadays, insulin pumps calculate IOB for you and deduct it, at least in part, from subsequent boluses (see Table 7-5). You might say that IOB is what puts the "smart" in today's smart pumps. By taking IOB into

Table 7-5. How different pumps handle IOB

Pump type	How it calculates IOB	What it does with IOB
Accu-Chek/Roche	Based only on correction boluses given, using a true curvilinear action profile	Calculates correction bolus required to reach predicted/desirable glucose level, based on time since bolus was given
Animas	Based on all boluses given, using a true curvilinear action profile	Deducts from correction bolus only if BG is above target
Deltec	Based on all boluses given, using linear action profile	Deducts full IOB from total correction plus meal dose if BG is below target
Insulet/OmniPod	Based only on correction boluses given, using a true curvilinear action profile	Deducts full IOB from total correction plus meal dose
Medtronic	Based on all boluses given, using a true curvilinear action profile	Deducts from correction bolus only

account, pumps make it safe to correct high readings at almost any time. However, different pumps have different ways of calculating IOB as well as applying it to bolus calculations. Should you trust the pump's IOB estimate? Will using it improve or hinder your control? Understanding how your pump handles IOB will help you answer these questions.

For those who don't own a smart pump or don't bother to use the pump's bolus calculator features, you will need to make the IOB adjustment on your own.

IOB should be based on the typical absorption and action patterns that you see when you take rapid-acting insulin. Keep in mind that insulin absorption and action can vary from person to person and from situation to situation. In some cases rapid insulin can be finished in just over two hours, and in other instances it can take as long as five or six. However, in most cases the actions of rapid-acting insulin follow the pattern shown in Figure 7-5 and Table 7-6.

Figure 7-5. Typical action profile of rapid-acting insulin

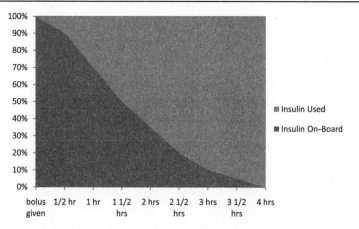

Table 7-6. IOB based on time since bolus was given.

Time since bolus was given	½ hour	1 hour	1½ hrs	2 hrs	2½ hrs	3 hrs	3½ hrs	4 hrs
Insulin used up	10%	30%	50%	65%	80%	90%	95%	100%
Insulin still on board	90%	70%	50%	35%	20%	10%	5%	0%

For example, if you gave yourself 6 units of insulin for a 3 p.m. snack and then check your blood sugar at 5 p.m., you still have 35 percent of your bolus remaining (6 units x .35 ≅ 2 units). If you gave 12 units at dinner and check your blood sugar three hours later, you still have approximately 1.2 units (12 x .10) remaining.

For the sake of simplicity, some people choose to assume that their insulin lasts a certain number of hours and figure a linear run-off of the insulin. Those who like to be aggressive with their dosing can assume a three-hour action time and figure that one-third of their insulin is used up each hour, as shown in Table 7-7.

Table 7-7. Simplified IOB based on three-hour action time

Time since bolus was given	1 hour	2 hours	3 hours
Insulin used up	33%	67%	100%
Insulin still on-board	67%	33%	0%

A more traditional approach assumes that the bolus takes four hours to finish working, and 25 percent is used up each hour. (See Table 7-8.)

Table 7-8. Simplified IOB based on four-hour action time

Time since bolus was given	1 hour	2 hours	3 hours	4 hours
Insulin used up	25%	50%	75%	100%
Insulin still on-board	75%	50%	25%	0%

For those who want to be more conservative with their dosing (in an effort to prevent hypoglycemia), assume that the insulin takes five hours to finish, and 20 percent is used up each hour.

Table 7-9. Simplified IOB based on five-hour action time

Time since bolus was given	1 hour	2 hours	3 hours	4 hours	5 hours
Insulin used up	20%	40%	60%	80%	100%
Insulin still on-board	80%	60%	40%	20%	0%

Figuring IOB More Precisely

Whether you use a pump to calculate your IOB or figure it out yourself, the calculation hinges on how long you think it takes for your insulin to finish working. You know what they say about people who make ASSumptions—so sometimes it's better to get the facts straight. Why? Because if you *underestimate* how long your insulin lasts, you will also underestimate how much IOB you have. And when you deduct too little IOB from your boluses, you open yourself up to more bouts of hypoglycemia. Conversely, if you *overestimate* how long your insulin lasts, you will also overestimate how much IOB you have. This can lead to excessive bolus deductions and more frequent hyperglycemia.

Confused yet? Don't worry. If you can determine your insulin action time properly, it won't matter.

There are a few ways to figure out how long it really takes for your bolus insulin to finish working. One way is to label your insulin with radioactive dye and see how long it takes for your body to stop glowing. Okay, maybe that's not all that practical. Another way is to check your blood sugar every thirty minutes after giving a correction bolus and then see how long it takes for the blood sugar to stop dropping. Once the correction bolus is given, you should not eat, exercise, or give any more boluses until you reach the point at which the blood sugar flattens out. Here is an example:

Time	Blood sugar
8 a.m.	238 mg/dl (13.2 mmol/l)
	✓ Correction bolus given
8:30	235 (13.1)
9:00	222 (12.3)
9:30	174 (9.8)
10:00	141 (7.8)
10:30	125 (6.9)
11:00	118 (6.6)
11:30	111 (6.2)
12:00 p.m.	112 (6.2)

It appears that the blood sugar flattened out at 11:30, which was three and a half hours after the bolus was given. So the duration of insulin action (also called "active insulin time") is three and a half hours.

A better way to measure how long it takes for your boluses to finish working (short of exposing yourself and your insulin to plutonium) is to watch the trend graph on a continuous glucose monitor after giving a correction bolus. Here are some examples:

Figure 7-6. Using CGM to determine insulin action time

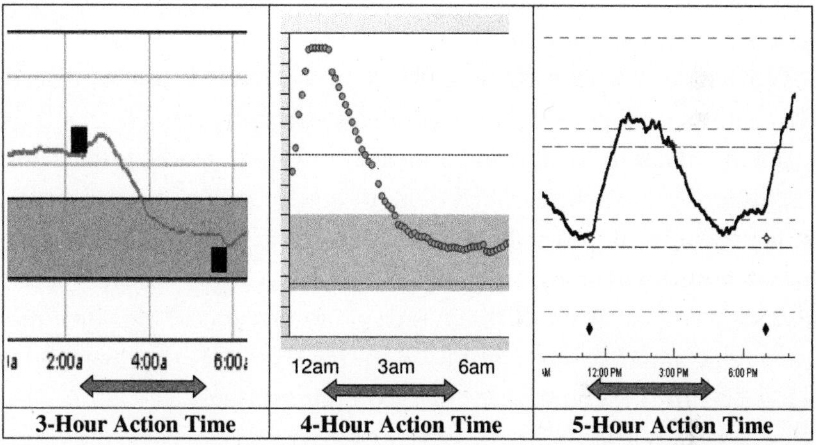

| 3-Hour Action Time | 4-Hour Action Time | 5-Hour Action Time |

In the example on the left, a correction bolus was given, and the blood sugar stopped falling after three hours. In the middle example, the correction bolus took four hours to finish. In the example on the right, a meal bolus was given, and the blood sugar stopped dropping at five hours.

What to Do with IOB

Regardless of the approach you use to calculate your IOB, taking IOB into account before giving any more boluses is very important. Whether you deduct IOB from correction boluses only or meal boluses as well is entirely up to you. Those who choose to deduct IOB only from correction boluses (i.e., high blood sugar doses) are assuming that any previous meal boluses are still covering undigested food. Although this may be true in some cases, the vast majority of carbohydrates digest pretty rapidly. That's why I prefer to deduct IOB from *any* boluses, whether they are being given to cover food, high blood sugar, or both.

However, if you recently had a meal or snack that you expect to digest slowly, only deducting IOB from correction boluses is reasonable because the original bolus is probably still offsetting undigested food. This includes times when you just had a very large quantity of food, a prolonged/drawn-out meal, or a meal consisting mainly of low-glycemic-index foods (these will be discussed later in this chapter under the subject of *Bolus Timing*).

Otherwise, simply subtract IOB from any bolus you plan to give. This helps to prevent stacking boluses and hypoglycemia. If you would normally take 4 units to cover a meal and/or high reading, but 1 unit is still active from an earlier bolus, it would be wise to give only 3 units. If you would normally take 2 units for an elevated blood sugar but 2.5 units are still active from a previous bolus, you should not take anything. In fact, if the IOB exceeds your correction bolus by a relatively large amount, you might need to snack in order to prevent a low blood sugar from occurring in the next couple hours.

(Food Dose + Correction Dose – Insulin On-Board)
x Activity Adjustment

Part 4. Adjustment for Physical Activity

Okay, let's see what we have so far. Bolus insulin is calculated based on the amount of carbohydrate, the blood sugar level, and the amount of insulin still working from previous boluses. So that's it, right? Well, not exactly.

You see, a unit of insulin is not always a unit of insulin. Let me put that another way: A unit of insulin given in one situation may work more or less effectively than a unit given in another situation. Something called *insulin sensitivity* determines insulin's effectiveness. The more sensitive we are to insulin, the more each unit will lower the blood sugar, and the more carbohydrate it will cover. A unit that normally lowers the blood sugar by 50 mg/dl (2.9 mmol/l) might lower it by 75 (4.4). A unit that usually covers 10 grams of carb might cover 15 or 20.

A number of factors can affect our sensitivity to insulin, but the most significant factor on a daily basis is physical activity. Not just exercise, but any form of physical activity, including cleaning, shopping, yard work, playing, sex, and anything else that has us using our muscles and breathing heavily.

Muscles are one of the main targets for insulin. With increased work, muscle cells become much more sensitive to insulin. This enhanced insulin sensitivity may continue for many hours, depending on the extent of the activity. The more intense and prolonged the activity, the longer and greater the enhancement in insulin sensitivity.

With enhanced insulin sensitivity, insulin exerts a greater force than usual. Thus, you will need to adjust boluses for upcoming and, in some cases, previous physical activity. Some forms of physical activity, most notably high-intensity/short-duration exercises and competitive sports, can produce a short-term rise in blood sugar levels. This is due primarily to an adrenaline surge. Adjustment for these types of activity will be discussed in the next chapter.

After-Meal Exercise

Most daily activities and aerobic exercises (exercises performed at a submaximal level over a period of twenty minutes or more) will cause blood sugar levels to drop due to enhanced insulin sensitivity and sugar metabolism. To prevent low blood sugar, you can reduce your insulin dose, increase your food intake, or both.

When exercise is going to be performed within two hours after a meal, the best approach is usually to reduce the mealtime bolus. Because physical activity influences both aspects of the bolus (the food part and the blood sugar correction part), both need to be reduced. To accomplish this, use an activity multiplier. Calculate your mealtime bolus as usual (based on the food, blood sugar level, and IOB) and then multiply the bolus by a factor that results in a dosage reduction (see Table 7-10).

Table 7-10. Bolus multipliers for physical activity

Activity multipliers	**Short** duration (15–30 minutes)	**Moderate** duration (40–60 minutes)	**Long** duration (>60 minutes)
Low intensity (RPE 8–11)	.90	.80	.70
Moderate intensity (RPE 12–15)	.75	.67	.50
High intensity (RPE 16–20)	.67	.50	.33

Exercise multipliers are based primarily on the duration and intensity of the activity. Whereas duration is fairly easy to measure, intensity is, shall we say, in the eye of the beholder. The "Rating of Perceived Exertion" chart in Figure 7-7 is a simple yet accurate way to assess the intensity of your workout. It takes into account the speed/pace of the activity, your current physical condition, number/size of muscles utilized, your skill/familiarity with the activity, and the workout environment.

For example, if Jan is planning a leisurely twenty-minute bike ride after dinner (she considers it "fairly light"), she would multiply her dinner bolus by .90, which would reduce her dose by 10 percent. If she plans a much more intense sixty-minute ride up and down hills (which she considers "very hard"), she would multiply her dinner dose by .50, which would reduce her dose by 50 percent.

Over time most of us experience a *conditioning effect*. This means that we tend to become more efficient at performing the same activity once we have had a chance to practice it. As a result, we burn less fuel and may require less of an insulin reduction. This also holds true for those who use food to prevent lows during exercise: Less food is required to maintain the blood sugar level as we become better conditioned.

Managing Pre-Activity Highs

Exercising with a high blood sugar level is rarely dangerous as long as there is at least a basal level of insulin in your body. Without a mini-

Figure 7–7. Rating of perceived exertion chart

Rating of perceived exertion scale (RPE)	
6	
7	Very, very light*
8	
9	Very light
10	
11	Fairly light
12	
13	Somewhat hard
14	
15	Hard
16	
17	Very hard
18	
19	Very, very hard*
20	

Very, very light activities constitute little more than resting, and typically do not require any insulin adjustments. Very, very hard activities (maximal intensity) are usually "anaerobic," meaning they cannot be performed for more than a few minutes and tend to cause a short-term rise in blood sugar levels.

mum level of insulin, exercise will cause the blood sugar to rise further and may accelerate the production of ketones, acidic by-products of fat metabolism. If ketones build up in large amounts and you become dehydrated, the delicate pH balance in the bloodstream and body tissues will become altered, and you will become susceptible to a life-threatening condition called diabetic ketoacidosis (DKA).

If your pre-exercise blood sugar is inexplicably high, there is one way to make sure you have sufficient insulin to allow for a safe exercise session: Check your urine (or your blood) for ketones. The presence of small, moderate, or large ketones in the urine, or a reading of greater than 0.5 mmol/l on a meter that measures ketones, indicates a lack of insulin in the body. Do not exercise if you have ketones; instead, drink plenty of water and contact your physician immediately.

If you do not have ketones, exercising should be safe as long as you address the high reading with insulin and drink plenty of water. However, high blood sugars during exercise can be a problem for anyone who wants to maximize their performance. As mentioned in Chapter 2, optimizing blood sugar levels during exercise can enhance your strength, speed, stamina, flexibility, and mental focus—all of which also add up to better athletic performance.

To treat high blood sugar prior to exercise, it is best to obtain a reading approximately thirty minutes before the activity. This will give the bolus insulin time to take effect before you start your activity. Because exercise has a tendency to amplify insulin's effects, you may only need a bolus that is half of what you would normally give to cover a high reading. For instance, if your normal sensitivity factor is 40 points per unit (2.2 mmol/l), assume an 80-point (4.4) drop per unit if you are about to exercise. If possible, test your blood sugar during and after your workout to see how well this works, adjusting as needed the next time around.

> For high blood sugar prior to exercise, take half the usual correction dose and drink plenty of water.

If you want to bring your blood sugar down as quickly as possible, consider giving the correction bolus by injection into a muscle rather than fat. An intramuscular injection can sting momentarily, but it will usually work twice as fast as an injection given into subcutaneous fat. Each unit given into muscle will have the same potency as a unit given into fat (i.e., lowers blood sugar the same amount), but it does so much faster.

Premeal Exercise

In some cases exercising before a meal will require a modest reduction in the bolus for the meal consumed *after* exercising. However, this is not usually necessary. If you notice that your blood sugar drops low after the meal following a workout, go ahead and reduce the bolus as needed.

In general, when exercise is going to be performed before or between meals, reducing the bolus at the previous meal would only drive the preworkout blood sugar very high. A better approach is to take the usual bolus at the previous meal and then snack prior to exercising. I will cover details regarding blood sugar management for premeal exercise in the next chapter, along with basal insulin adjustments for prolonged and exhaustive forms of exercise.

Inactivity: Sensitivity in Reverse

What goes up, must come down. Just as increased physical activity causes an improvement in insulin sensitivity, decreased activity can have the opposite effect. Anyone who has gone from a physical job to a sedentary one, or an active lifestyle to prolonged recuperation from an injury, knows what this is all about.

Any time you are very *inactive* at a time when you are normally active, your insulin is not going to work as well as usual. For example, this can happen when you spend several hours or more

- sitting in meetings;
- sitting in planes, trains, or automobiles;
- sitting at a show;
- working at a desk;
- working in front of the computer;
- napping;
- watching TV;
- playing video games; or
- reading.

Long periods of inactivity create a temporary state of insulin resistance so more insulin is required to get the same job done. When this happens, consider taking your bolus doses *up* in small increments—perhaps using a bolus multiplier of 1.1 (a 10 percent increase), 1.2 (20 percent increase) or 1.25 (25 percent increase).

For example, let's say Armond is about to board a three-hour flight to Cleveland to visit the Rock and Roll Hall of Fame. Before giving his usual lunch bolus of 5 units, he multiplies the dose by 1.2 and gives 6 units instead. Rock on!

(Food Dose + Correction Dose – Insulin On-Board)
x Activity Adjustment

Part 5. Bolus Timing

Let's see . . . so far, we've learned about key dimensions to figuring out a bolus: the part that covers food, the part that covers the blood sugar, and adjustments for insulin on-board and physical activity. These dimensions should just about do the job—unless you live in the real world, where the fourth dimension, time, is of the essence.

The timing of your boluses can make or break their effectiveness. To understand this concept, imagine yourself as a baseball player, batting against a very clever pitcher. Not only do you have to swing the bat at the level where the ball is, but you also have to swing it at the right time—when the ball is just crossing the plate. If you swing too early or too late, all you'll hear is the sound of the ball hitting the catcher's mitt and the umpire yelling, "STEEEERIKE!" Likewise, boluses must be timed properly. Even if the *amount* of the bolus is correct, giving it too early will cause a low blood sugar followed by high readings several hours later. Boluses given too late will produce significant hyperglycemia soon after eating. A properly timed bolus in the proper quantity . . . now, there's a thing of beauty. (Excuse me . . . I'm getting all misty just thinking about it—sniff!)

The only assumption is that you will be using a rapid-acting analog (aspart, glulisine, or lispro) for your boluses. If you are still using regular insulin (or a premixed insulin that contains regular insulin), take all the advice given below and back it up twenty to thirty minutes.

In order to achieve optimal control of your blood sugar for the first couple hours after eating, the timing of your boluses should be based on a few key variables: the type of food you will be eating, your premeal blood sugar level, and the presence or absence of impaired digestion.

Glycemic Index

The glycemic index (GI) tells us how rapidly food raises the blood sugar level. Although virtually all carbohydrates convert into blood sugar eventually, some forms do so much faster than others. Pure glucose is given a GI score of 100; everything else is compared to the digestion/absorption rate of glucose. See Appendix C for GI listings for many common foods.

Most starchy foods have a relatively high GI; this means that they digest easily and convert into blood sugar quickly. Some starches, such as legumes (beans, nuts) and pasta digest quite slowly. Foods that have dextrose in them tend to have a very high GI. Table sugar (sucrose) has a moderate GI, whereas fructose (fruit sugar) and lactose (milk sugar) are somewhat slower at raising blood sugar. Foods that contain fiber or large amounts of fat tend to have lower GIs than comparable foods that do not. For example, French fries tend to raise the blood sugar more slowly than baked potatoes do, and apples tend to be a bit slower than apple juice. See Figure 7-8 for a summary of how glycemic index affects the timing and magnitude of the postmeal blood sugar rise.

Figure 7-8. Blood sugar rise based on glycemic index

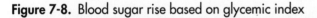
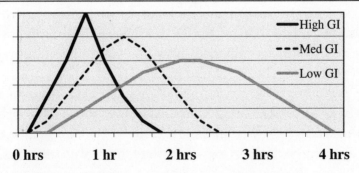

Foods with a high GI (greater than 70) tend to raise blood sugar the fastest, with a significant peak occurring in about thirty to forty-five minutes. Examples include bread, potatoes, cereal, white rice, and sugary candies. For these types of foods, *you should bolus twenty to thirty minutes prior to eating*. Doing so will allow the insulin peak to coincide as closely as possible with the blood sugar peak. And that, of course, will produce the best after-meal control. Bolusing for high-GI foods just before, during, or after eating is not ideal. The food will raise the blood sugar long before the insulin kicks in, thereby producing a significant after-meal blood sugar spike followed by a pronounced drop. If you are not sure how much you are going to eat, bolus for an amount that you are confident you will have and then give the rest when the meal is over. That way most of your bolus insulin will be on the job when you need it most.

Foods with a moderate GI (approximately 45–69) digest a bit slower, resulting in a more modest blood sugar peak approximately sixty to ninety minutes after eating. Examples include ice cream, orange juice, cake, and carrots. Bolusing thirty minutes before eating these types of foods could produce a low blood sugar soon after eating. You should bolus five to ten minutes prior to moderate GI foods.

Foods with a low GI (below 45) tend to produce a slow, gradual blood sugar rise. The blood sugar peak is usually modest and may take several hours to appear. Examples include whole-grain pasta, milk, yogurt, beans, and chocolate. The same slow, gradual blood sugar rise occurs when consuming meals or snacks over an extended period of time (such as holiday meals, popcorn, or party food) or having very large portions. In these situations bolusing prior to eating tends to produce a blood sugar drop followed by a marked rise a few hours later as the bolus wears off and food starts to take its effect. Instead, try these options when having slow-digesting foods:

- Bolus soon after eating. This usually gives the food enough of a head start before the insulin kicks in.
- Split the bolus into two parts: half given with the meal and the remainder given one to two hours later. Wearing a watch

with an alarm can help remind you to give the second half of the bolus.

- Take regular insulin with the meal rather than a rapid-acting insulin analog. With its delayed peak and prolonged action, regular insulin does a better job of matching the blood sugar rise from low-GI foods.
- If you use an insulin pump, use a combination or dual-wave bolus, with 25 to 33 percent of the bolus delivered immediately with the meal and the remainder delivered gradually over two hours.

For a summary of bolus timing based on glycemic index, see Table 7-10.

Table 7-11. Optimal bolus timing based on glycemic index of food

High-GI food	Bolus well before eating
Moderate-GI food	Bolus soon before eating
Low-GI food, prolonged or very large meals	Bolus after eating, or spread out delivery

Blood Sugar

The second major variable to consider when determining the optimal timing of your boluses is the premeal blood sugar level. To avoid an after-meal blood sugar spike or major drop, you should give the bolus earlier, when the blood sugar is elevated, and again later when the blood sugar is below your target range. Table 7-12 summarizes optimal bolus timing based on glycemic index and premeal blood sugar.

Table 7-12. Adjustments to bolus timing based on GI and premeal blood sugar

Bolus timing in relation to meal ⬋	High GI	Moderate GI	Low GI, prolonged or large meal
BG above target	35–45 min. prior	20–25 min. prior	0–10 min. prior
BG within target	20–30 min. prior	5–10 min. prior	5–15 min. after
BG below target	0–15 min. prior	5–10 min. after	20–30 min. after

When Will It Digest?
What If I'm Still Spiking after Meals?

If you are timing your boluses properly but your after-meal blood sugar is still above acceptable levels, don't give up. There are a number of very effective strategies that you can use to "Strike the Spike." I will present these in detail in Chapter 9.

Put It All Together

(Food Dose + Correction Dose − Insulin On-Board)
x Activity Adjustment

⏲ TIMED PROPERLY ⏲
=

The *Ultimate* Bolus!!!
Congratulations!!!

Chapter Highlights

- Bolus doses should be based on four things: carbs, blood sugar, activity, and insulin on-board.
- Insulin-to-carb ratios allow you to adjust your dose to match your exact food intake.
- Correction doses are based on your precise target blood sugar and your sensitivity to each unit of insulin
- Deducting insulin on-board (insulin still working from recent boluses) from your boluses will help prevent hypoglycemia.
- Increased physical activity will usually require a percentage reduction in your usual bolus dose. Decreased activity may require a modest dosage increase.
- Frequent blood sugar testing/record keeping and using CGM can help you and your health care team fine-tune your bolus dosing.
- Proper timing of boluses is necessary to obtain the best after-meal control.

CHAPTER 8

Welcome to
the Real World

So there you are: Armed with a physiologically perfect basal insulin program and a set of bolus equations that would impress your old, crotchety high school algebra teacher, off you go to conquer your favorite Italian restaurant.

There's going to be a half-hour wait for a table. "No problem," you say to yourself. "My basal insulin should take care of that." Well, thanks to a huge party that just won't leave, that thirty-minute wait turns into sixty minutes. Irritated, you start walking past the table, clearing your throat as loudly as possible. No movement . . . time to hit the bar.

As time ticks away, the Diet Cokes turn into rum and Diet Cokes. Finally, the hostess calls out your name (mispronounced, but close enough). Elation quickly turns to frustration as she brings your party of four to a table for two. "I asked for a table for four," you tell her.

"Are you sure? Well, I'll have to see what we have available." You can feel the veins in your head starting to swell.

Fifteen minutes later your group finds its way to a table for four. Your frustration grows once again as you check your blood sugar to find that it has risen a great deal since you left home. "I haven't eaten a thing . . . how could this happen?" you ask yourself. Oh well, nothing a little extra insulin can't fix.

Your meal features the usual array of breadsticks, salad with rich dressing, pasta with cream sauce, and cheesecake for dessert. Counting your carbs as carefully as possible, you bolus the exact amount your bolus formulas dictate. You even give the insulin *after* your meal because it contains a lot of slow-digesting foods—something you remembered reading about in Chapter 7. This is a plan that can't possibly fail, right?

Wrong. On the way out of the restaurant, you start feeling a bit woozy. No problem—you whip out your trusty meter, smear on some blood, and it reads: "low." Now you're really confused. How could you possibly be low after a meal like that? No matter, grab a handful of mints from the hostess stand (it's the least they could do after making you wait so long!) and let someone else drive home.

Hopefully, all is not lost. You did count your carbs and bolus the right amount, so your bedtime reading should be decent. In fact, it is only slightly above target, but given all you had to eat, that's not so bad. A minor insulin touch-up, and it's off to sleep.

That night, you have a nightmare about a giant lasagna chasing you with a fork. To make matters worse, you have to get up several times during the night to pee. Upon waking the next morning, you discover that your blood sugar isn't just up—it's *way* up. "That's it," you tell yourself. "I'm never going to *that* restaurant again. From now on, nothing but home cookin'."

Welcome to the real world, where things hardly ever go as planned, and blood sugars don't always turn out as expected.

In Chapter 3, we concentrated on the major factors that influence blood sugar levels: insulin and other diabetes medications, food (specifically carbohydrates), physical activity, and the liver's secretion of glucose. We spent the next several chapters focusing on how to set up the insulin program and adjust doses to match those factors. Now it's time to pay homage to the secondary factors: those pesky day-to-day oddities that tend to mess with good control.

The Other Stuff That Can *Raise* Blood Sugar

Anxiety/Stress

Anxious moments and nerve-racking situations happen to all of us. From speaking in public to test taking to a simple visit to the doctor or dentist—

many events elicit a stress hormone response that causes, among other things, a sharp blood sugar rise. To the right in Figure 8-1 is a CGM readout showing a dramatic blood sugar rise I once experienced when I was late for an important meeting, hit a pothole and got a flat tire, and then discovered that the spare tire was also flat. Without the slightest bit of food, my blood sugar rose almost 300 mg/dl (17 mmol/l)!

Figure 8-1. CGM printout showing a stress response

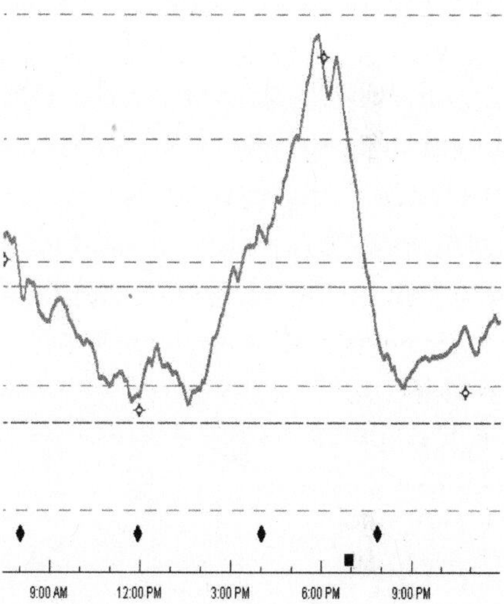

Of course, different events cause different responses in different people. What causes a great deal of anxiety for you might have no effect on someone else. The key is to look for patterns. Is there something that causes a consistent blood sugar response in a given situation? It can be helpful to record the *causes* of your high blood sugars in your written records and then tally the causes to determine whether specific situations account for a large number of high readings. One of my clients did this and found that high blood sugars were occurring every time he watched a horror movie. Apparently, the stress hormone response to the sudden appearances of the knife-wielding maniac was driving his blood sugar up.

> If you can predict it, you can usually prevent it.

The Adjustment: Many anxious moments occur spontaneously. However, some can be predicted—and if you can predict it, you can prevent it. If you notice a consistent pattern of high blood sugars with certain events, consider giving yourself a small dose of rapid-acting insulin an hour or two prior to the event. This will help to offset the stress hormones produced in anticipation of the event as well as during the event itself. If you wear an insulin pump, consider raising your basal rate by using the temp basal feature. A 60 to 80 percent increase for three hours, starting one to two hours prior to the event, can work nicely.

The first time you try the adjustment, be certain to check your blood sugar frequently to see how well the extra insulin is working. A student I work with tends to run very high blood sugars when taking standardized tests in school. Her parents agreed to give her extra insulin at breakfast on the mornings of standardized testing, and her blood sugar turned out to be very close to normal at lunchtime. And who knows? Keeping your blood sugar near normal might enable you to cope better with the stressful situation.

Caffeine

A natural stimulant, caffeine tends to cause a rise in blood sugar levels in approximately one hour. It does this by promoting the breakdown of fat (rather than sugar) for energy and stimulating the liver's breakdown of glycogen. Granted, the amount of caffeine found in most foods is insignificant. However, consumption of large amounts of caffeine can produce a noticeable blood sugar rise. Below is a list of some of the major sources of caffeine:

Jolt energy drink: 280 mg
stay-awake pills: 100–200 mg
Monster energy drink: 160 mg
5-Hour energy drink: 138 mg
brewed coffee (8 oz): 100–120 mg
espresso: 100 mg

latte: 100 mg
Red Bull: 80 mg
instant coffee (8 oz): 60–80 mg
tea (8 oz): 30–50 mg
cola (12 oz): 30–45 mg
cold tablets: 30 mg
chocolate bar: 20–30 mg
chocolate milk (12 oz): 10 mg

The Adjustment: If you suspect that caffeine may be causing your blood sugar to rise, either look for a lower-caffeine substitute or take a little extra rapid-acting insulin when consuming high-caffeine foods/ beverages. To determine the amount of insulin you need, test your blood sugar and then consume the caffeinated item with no other food (bolus only for the carbs in the caffeinated item). Check your blood sugar again in three hours and then divide the rise by your sensitivity factor. For example, if a sixteen-ounce coffee makes your blood sugar rise by about 80 mg/dl (4.4 mmol/l) and your sensitivity factor is 40 mg/dl (2.2 mmol/l), you need to take 2 units of insulin just to offset the effects of the caffeine in the coffee.

Disease Progression

Most people with type 1 diabetes as well as LADA go through a "honeymoon" phase soon after diagnosis. For several weeks, months, or even years the pancreas continues to produce a small amount of insulin. This results in blood glucose levels that are stable and near normal, particularly overnight and first thing in the morning. Usually, the pancreas first loses the ability to secrete sufficient amounts of bolus insulin. Then the ability to produce basal insulin begins to fade. As a result, blood sugars become higher and more erratic, particularly upon waking in the morning. Likewise, type 2 diabetes becomes progressively more difficult to manage as the body becomes more insulin-resistant and the pancreas loses the ability to produce sufficient amounts of insulin.

The Adjustment: For those with type 1 diabetes or LADA who are exiting the honeymoon, fasting (or morning) blood sugars will tend to be elevated—perhaps for the first time ever. You will need increases in basal insulin in order to manage overnight blood sugar levels. You may also eventually need increases in bolus doses as the pancreas loses its ability to produce basal insulin throughout the day. For those with type 2 diabetes, the gradual loss of insulin-producing beta cells means that insulin dosage requirements will gradually increase. If you experience blood sugars that are above target for three days in a row, it is time to increase the insulin dose at the preceding meal (or the basal insulin dose, if the high readings occurred first thing in the morning).

Protein

For many years nutrition experts believed that dietary protein caused blood sugar to rise. Then studies of mixed meals (meals containing carbs, protein, and fat) showed that protein had no effect. So what are we to believe? In cases like this, I prefer to rely on experience. What we see time and again is that protein does, in fact, raise blood sugar, but only when consumed without carbohydrates. Roughly 50 percent of protein can be converted to glucose if there is no other source of sugar in the meal. Carbohydrates have a "sparing" effect on this process. This means that when carbs are eaten, protein is used for purposes other than supplying blood sugar, such as bodily growth, repair, and creating hormones and enzymes, but without carbs protein becomes a source of glucose for nourishing the body's cells.

The Adjustment: If you have no carbs in a meal or snack, count up the grams of protein that you are consuming. (See Table 8-1.) Take half that amount and bolus for it as if it was carbohydrate. Of course, if the protein amount is very modest (for example, a slice of cheese), the effect on the blood sugar will hardly be noticeable, so you will not need to bolus.

Things get a bit trickier, however, if your meal or snack contains protein and only a small amount of carbohydrate. If the carbohydrate

Table 8-1. Protein content of protein-rich foods

1 ounce of beef, pork, or fish	7g protein
1 ounce of poultry	9g protein
1 large egg	6g protein
1 cup milk	8g protein
½ cup cottage cheese	15g protein
1 ounce cheese	8g protein
½ cup ice cream	3g protein
½ cup tofu	20g protein
½ cup cooked beans	8g protein
¼ cup peanuts	9g protein
¼ cup seeds	7g protein
2 tablespoons peanut butter	8g protein

is insufficient to meet the body's need for glucose, some of the protein may be converted to glucose. Having at least a moderate amount of carbohydrate in each meal and snack is usually a good idea. That way, the effects of protein on blood sugar can basically be ignored.

Fatty Foods

Consuming large amounts of fat in a meal or snack can cause blood sugar levels to rise in a gradual manner over a period of six to ten hours or more. This delayed rise is in addition to the immediate rise carbohydrates cause. The mechanism by which fat causes a delayed rise in the blood sugar is not entirely understood, but it is believed to be the result of insulin resistance. When you consume a high-fat meal, the level of triglycerides in your bloodstream rises. This sends your liver into a temporary state of insulin resistance, resulting in greater secretion of glucose into the bloodstream.

Although there is no specific amount of fat that causes a delayed blood sugar rise in everybody, having more than 20 grams of fat certainly increases the likelihood that a delayed rise will occur. Some foods commonly associated with high fat content and delayed blood sugar rises are listed below.

- Restaurant foods: Meals prepared at restaurants usually have a great deal of fat added during preparation.
- Take-out food: pizza = 10–20 g fat per slice; hot wings = 2–3 g each; Chinese food: egg roll = 15 g, fried rice = 13 g/cup, sweet and sour pork = 25 g/cup.
- Fast food: small cheeseburger = 15 g fat; Big Mac = 30 g; average taco = 11 g; sausage/egg/cheese sandwich = 40 g.
- Fried foods: oils used in preparing fried food contain 10–15 g fat per tablespoon; fried fish sandwich = 23 g; fried chicken patty = 14 g; small order of French fries =15 g.
- High-fat meats: most cuts of beef, lamb, pork, dark meat chicken/turkey, and sardines contain approximately 8–15 g fat per three ounces (a deck of cards–sized serving); ground round/hamburger = 20 g; ribs and sausage = 25 g; most lunch meats = 10 g per slice; a hot dog = 15 g.
- Cheesy dishes: approximately 70 percent of cheese is pure fat; American/cheddar/Swiss cheese = 8–10 g per ounce (or slice); mozzarella/parmesan = 6–7 g per ounce.
- Dessert items: an average slice of chocolate cake = 15 g fat; ice cream = 10–15 g per half-cup; a cinnamon bun = 25 g; 1 doughnut, muffin, slice of cake, or chocolate bar = 10–20 g; 1 slice apple pie or cheesecake = 20 g.
- Salty snacks: chips = 10 g fat per handful; peanuts = 10–15 g per small handful; a medium movie-theater popcorn = 60 g fat (without butter topping); nachos with cheese = 20–30 g.

Each person needs to determine based on their own experience how much fat he or she requires to produce a delayed blood sugar rise. For example, I find that a single slice of pizza rarely causes my blood sugar to rise after the first couple of hours. However, after eating two or more slices I usually see a significant rise over the next six to eight hours.

The Adjustment: As was the case with stress responses, if you can predict it, you can prevent it. When a delayed rise in blood sugar is anticipated, two options are available. For those taking insulin by injection, intermediate-acting insulin (NPH) tends to do a nice job of offsetting the effects of fat. Taking a small dose of intermediate insulin along with your rapid-acting mealtime insulin provides a nice one-two punch: The rapid insulin covers the immediate rise produced by the carbohydrates, and the intermediate insulin covers the delayed rise produced by the fat. A dose of NPH equal to 5 to 10 percent of your total daily insulin should serve as a safe starting point. For example, if you average a total of 50 units of insulin for the day (basal + bolus combined), give yourself 2.5 to 5 units of NPH with a high-fat meal.

If you are using an insulin pump, the adjustment is much simpler. Try a temporary basal increase of 50 to 60 percent lasting approximately eight hours, starting after you finish your meal. Check your blood sugar frequently the first time you do this to see how well the adjustment is working.

Growth and Weight Gain

During a young person's growth years insulin needs rise steadily. This is due to increases in the production of hormones, which counteract insulin and stimulate the liver to produce additional glucose as well as increases in body size. The accumulation of body fat also increases insulin requirements because fat cells secrete hormones that cause insulin resistance.

The Adjustment: All aspects of the insulin program will need to increase with significant growth and weight gain. Adjustments should be made in proportion to the amount of weight gained or lost. With a 10 percent change in body mass, changes are usually needed in basal insulin levels, insulin-carb ratios, and the sensitivity factor. For example, a person who goes from 120 to 130 pounds (57 to 62 kg) and has blood sugars that are consistently above his or her target range should consider increasing basal, bolus, and correction insulin by approximately 10 percent.

Illness/Infection

Infections are more common in people with diabetes, particularly when blood sugar levels are chronically high. Infection-fighting white blood cells do not work well when the blood sugar is elevated. Extra glucose in the bloodstream also provides nourishment for viruses and bacteria (aiding and abetting the enemy!). Infections, in turn, cause the body to produce stress hormones that drive the blood sugar even higher and make insulin less effective.

Infections commonly affect the sinuses, respiratory system, urinary and vaginal tract, and skin. Symptoms of infection include:

- chronically high blood sugars
- fever
- dehydration
- enlarged glands
- thick yellow, green, or milky secretions

Ketones may be present in the blood and urine during an illness and this is caused by insulin's lack of effectiveness (as a result of all the stress hormones that are being produced). It is important to check your blood sugar and ketones frequently during an illness and stay in close contact with your health care team.

The Adjustment: Even if you are not eating as much as usual, be sure to keep taking your basal insulin during an illness. Without basal insulin, your blood sugar will go dangerously high and you will put yourself at risk of diabetic ketoacidosis (DKA). When in DKA, your blood becomes so acidic that you will likely be vomiting and extremely achy. Your breathing will become very deep and labored, and your breath will take on a characteristic spoiled-fruit smell as your lungs attempt to rid your body of acid when you exhale. Treatment for DKA requires an immediate trip to your nearest emergency room.

In most cases extra basal insulin is required during an illness. If your blood sugars are repeatedly high and you are *not* ketotic, consider increasing your basal insulin dose by 25 to 50 percent. If you are ketotic (small or more on a urine ketostick, or >0.5 on a blood meter that measures ketones), increase the basal insulin 50 to 100 percent. The basal insulin increase is in addition to your usual bolus doses, including correction doses to cover high blood sugars.

Keep in mind that insulin will not absorb properly into the bloodstream if you are not adequately hydrated. Drinking plenty of fluids during an illness is essential—preferably clear, caffeine-free fluids. Most adults should consume one cup per hour while awake; small children should consume a half cup per hour. If you suspect that your insulin is not working after you inject or bolus into the fat below the skin, consider giving an injection directly into muscle or ask to be taken to a hospital so that insulin and fluids may be administered intravenously.

Couch Potato Syndrome

Sitting for long periods of time when you are normally active can produce a gradual rise in the blood sugar level. Because your usual insulin doses are based on a standard level of physical activity, withdrawing that activity can result in less glucose burning and a temporary decrease in insulin sensitivity.

The Adjustment: The next time you plan to be completely sedentary for more than a few hours, consider raising your insulin dose slightly. If you use a pump, a temporary basal increase of 40 percent is a good place to start. If you take injections, adding 20 or 30 percent to your boluses can do the job nicely. Try this the next time you take a long car trip or plane/train/bus ride as well as any time you plan to veg out in front of the TV, the computer, or a good book for several hours.

Rebounds from Lows/Somogyi Phenomenon

A "rebound" may cause the high readings that follow hypoglycemic episodes. The symptoms that accompany low blood sugars (especially shaking, sweating, and rapid heartbeat) are caused by the production of adrenaline, and not surprisingly, adrenaline can also raise the blood sugar and inhibit insulin's action for the next several hours. This can cause the blood sugar level to be unusually high and makes it difficult to bring down with your usual dose of correction insulin.

When low blood sugars occur during sleep, the body's own natural hormonal responses commonly kick in and produce high readings upon waking. This is referred to as a Somogyi Phenomenon. Many people sleep through these mild lows and are surprised to see the high readings when they wake up. Many believe that they need more insulin overnight to control the morning highs. Of course, increasing the nighttime insulin would only make the problem worse!

The following symptoms may indicate that you are going low and rebounding during the night:

- nighttime sweating
- cool body temperature
- restlessness
- headache/hangover-like symptoms
- rapid heartbeat upon waking
- strange dreams
- not feeling well rested in the morning

It is a good idea to periodically check your blood sugar at the midpoint of your sleep time to verify that your blood sugar is not dropping while you sleep. If getting up in the middle of the night doesn't appeal to you, try wearing a continuous glucose monitor and check the trend graphs when you wake up in the morning. For example, the chart in Figure 8-2 indicates consistent blood sugar drops in the middle of the night, followed by a rise in the early morning:

The Adjustment: When morning highs are preceded by lows in the middle of the night, there are a number of possible solutions.

1. If the lows are always preceded by highs at bedtime, increase your sensitivity factor starting after dinner. That way you will receive less insulin to cover bedtime highs.

Figure 8-2. CGM printout showing nighttime low blood sugars followed by wake-up highs

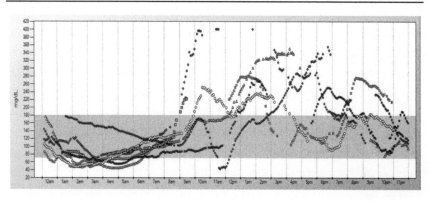

2. If the lows are more common after large bedtime snacks, reduce your insulin-to-carb ratio for food eaten after dinner.

3. If the lows take place when no bolus was given at bedtime, reduce the basal insulin from bedtime to morning (if using a pump) or the dose of long-acting insulin (if taking injections).

Unfortunately, predicting when—or if—a rebound is going to occur after typical garden-variety hypoglycemic episodes is difficult. If you experience a consistent rebound at a consistent time following lows (or certain types of lows), giving a dose of insulin designed to prevent the rise is reasonable. For example, if your blood sugar always rebounds to the 300s (17–22 mmol/l) in the afternoon following pre-lunch lows, you might consider taking extra insulin at lunchtime. If you consistently rebound to very high levels two to three hours after readings below 50 (2.2), you might consider taking a small dose of rapid-acting insulin (or raising your basal rate for a few hours if you wear a pump) after you have treated the low.

Speaking of treatment, another way to prevent a significant rebound is to refrain from overtreating the low. Eating excessive amounts of food when you are low is like throwing gasoline on a fire. I will discuss proper treatment of lows in the next chapter.

Steroids

Steroidal medications such as cortisone and prednisone are used to treat asthma, arthritis, emphysema, and muscle/joint inflammation. These drugs create significant insulin resistance and raise blood sugar levels—sometimes dramatically. Inhalers (containing albuterol) and topical steroids (in cream or ointment form) can also raise blood sugar levels. For those using a steroid medication on an ongoing basis, increasing the steroid dose can lead to blood sugars that are higher than usual.

The Adjustment: Some steroids are more potent than others, and their onset/duration of action can vary. Ask your physician about the specific medication that you plan to use. In most cases single doses of a steroid medication (for example, an injection of cortisone for knee, shoulder, or elbow inflammation) will raise the blood sugar for anywhere from six to forty-eight hours. You may need to increase your basal insulin by as much as 50 to 300 percent until the steroid wears off.

Other Medications

Diuretics, Dilantin, estrogen, testosterone, epinephrine, and cough/cold remedies that contain epinephrine, certain antibiotics (fluoroquinolone versions), lithium, and many beta blockers can cause a short-term rise in blood sugar levels. Thyroid medications (taken by those with an underactive thyroid gland) can also induce a modest elevation.

The Adjustment: If you have been taking any of these medications over an extended period of time, no insulin dosage adjustments should be necessary. However, if you are starting or increasing a dose, you may need to increase the insulin bolus given after taking the medication. In the case of thyroid medication, you may need to make changes to your basal insulin when starting or increasing a dose.

Surgery

Medical procedures, ranging from oral surgery to a tummy tuck to cardiac bypass, have certain physiological and psychological consequences. Among these is a stress response by the body (in response to an invasion by "foreign fingers") as well as the mind (in anticipation of the event). There is also a recovery period that involves bed rest and a certain degree of discomfort. What's it all mean for your diabetes? Yep, high blood sugars—and at the worst possible time. A speedy recovery hinges on good blood sugar control. The body's tissues heal better and with less risk of infection when the blood sugar is near normal.

The Adjustment: If your surgeon offers to control your blood sugars for you during and after the procedure, take her up on it. The medical team will monitor your blood sugar frequently and infuse insulin directly into your bloodstream via an IV to keep your blood sugar as close to normal as possible.

For outpatient procedures your doctor will probably ask you to manage your own diabetes. That's okay—it's not as complicated as it may seem. Because most procedures require you to fast beforehand, surgeons will typically schedule their patients with diabetes first thing in the morning. (Take advantage of it! We might as well get something for having this disease!)

Even though you won't be eating beforehand, you may need extra basal insulin to offset the effects of stress hormones prior to and during the procedure as well as lack of activity (and discomfort) after the procedure. You should give bolus insulin if/when your blood sugar is elevated. Here's a quick guide to help you manage.

If you use an insulin pump: Stay connected to the pump before, during, and after the procedure. However, make sure your infusion set and tubing will not get in the surgeon's way. Keep your basal insulin at the *normal level.* Reducing your basal will almost certainly cause your blood sugar to run quite high. Cover your presurgery blood sugar with a standard correction bolus, and bolus as usual for your after-surgery meals/snacks. Following the procedure, if you find that your blood sugar remains elevated for more than a few hours, consider raising your basal by 50 percent by using the temp basal feature.

If you take glargine, detemir, or NPH (at night): Take your usual dose of basal insulin. An hour or two prior to the procedure check your blood

sugar and administer a correction bolus as needed. After the procedure check again and bolus as needed.

If you take NPH in the morning: Give 50 percent of your usual dose of
NPH the morning of the procedure. Include a dose of rapid-acting insulin if you wake up with high blood sugar. Cover all meals during the
day (including lunch) with rapid insulin. If you are unable to eat, test
your blood sugar every two to three hours and administer correction
insulin as needed.

The Other Stuff That Can *Lower* Blood Sugar

Prior Heavy Exercise

Have you ever finished a workout with a terrific blood sugar only to go
low, out of the blue, hours later? *Delayed-onset hypoglycemia* (or D'OH,
as Homer Simpson likes to say) is a blood sugar drop that occurs several hours after a high-intensity, long-duration, or exhaustive workout.
It typically occurs six to twelve hours afterward, but it can take place
up to twenty-four to forty-eight hours later. The timing of the drop
varies from person to person and sport to sport. In my own case, playing full-court basketball in the evening usually results in a blood sugar
drop the next morning before lunch.

There are two reasons why delayed blood sugar drops take place.
Heavy exercise makes muscle cells very sensitive to insulin, so following physical activity every unit of insulin will cover a greater amount
of carbohydrate and have a greater blood sugar–lowering effect. Exhaustive exercise can also deplete the glycogen (sugar energy stores)
in the muscles and liver, and as muscle and liver cells replenish their
glycogen stores, blood sugar levels tend to drop.

The Adjustment: The first step in dealing with D'OH is to determine
when it happens and under what circumstances. Keeping detailed written records should allow you to figure out which types of activities induce a delayed drop as well as the timing. For example, since learning
that nighttime basketball makes my blood sugar drop the next day at

midmorning, I started reducing my breakfast bolus the morning after full-court hoops.

So once again, if you can predict it, you can prevent it. Strategies for preventing D'OH include:

- reducing your pump's basal insulin leading up to the time of the expected blood sugar drop,
- lowering the bolus at the meal preceding the expected drop,
- reducing the long-acting insulin that will be active at the time of the expected drop, and
- having a slow-digesting snack prior to the time of the expected drop.

Weight Loss

Just as weight gain increases insulin needs, weight loss reduces it. Losing as little as five pounds (2.4 kg) can enhance your insulin sensitivity and improve the overall effectiveness of your insulin.

The Adjustment: All aspects of the insulin program will need to be adjusted with weight loss: basal insulin, insulin-carb ratios, and the sensitivity factor. For those trying to lose weight, reducing insulin doses as the weight begins to come off is absolutely necessary. Otherwise, repeated bouts of hypoglycemia will hinder further weight loss efforts. For example, someone who goes from 240 to 230 pounds (114 to 109 kg) and begins to experience below-target blood sugars should reduce his or her doses by 5 to 10 percent across the board.

Aging

With advanced age comes a reduction in hormones (such as growth hormone) that counteract insulin and stimulate the liver's release of glucose.

The Adjustment: Be prepared to cut back on basal insulin levels after age sixty. Hypoglycemia is particularly dangerous in the elderly due to impaired counter-regulation—the body's hormones do little to help raise the blood sugar back toward normal in the event of a low—as well as the risk of falls and heart attacks when hypoglycemia strikes.

Brain Work

The central nervous system is one of the body's major consumers of glucose. Brain cells rely almost exclusively on glucose for energy. Whenever the brain is working hard, blood sugar levels may drop. This can occur during periods of intense concentration (studying, multi-tasking), adjustment to new surroundings (new job, new home), and complex social situations (hosting a party, business networking, "working the floor"). Simply being in an environment that features lots of mental stimulation, such as a shopping center, supermarket, arcade, or casino, can make blood sugars drop.

The Adjustment: Predicting when brain activity is going to be high enough to induce a blood sugar drop can be difficult. (In fact, trying to figure it out constitutes brain activity itself!) If you detect a pattern of blood sugar drops in certain situations, either reducing your insulin or increasing your food intake in anticipation of such events makes sense.

For example, I have a tendency to "drop while I shop" at the supermarket. In response, I try to go grocery shopping after dinner (real men shop at night) and then reduce my dinner bolus by about a third to prevent hypoglycemia. If I forget to make the adjustment, I'll just graze on a few pretzel sticks while I shop.

Climate

Warm temperature and humidity have a tendency to cause blood sugar levels to drop. This is caused by heightened energy expenditure by the circulatory and respiratory systems as well as accelerated absorption of insulin from below the skin.

The Adjustment: Seasonal changes may require modest (10 to 20 percent) changes in basal as well as bolus insulin doses. You may need short-term dosage adjustments when traveling to a climate that is warmer or more humid than what you are used to. When you move exercise from indoors to outdoors you may require a more significant preworkout bolus reduction than usual, particularly when the weather outside is very hot or humid. When taking injections of long-acting/basal insulin, try to inject into areas that will not be heated excessively by shower/bath water within a few hours of the injection; otherwise, the insulin may absorb and run out faster than desired.

High Altitude

Traveling to altitudes that are much higher than you are accustomed to can cause blood sugar levels to drop. At high altitudes the metabolism (heart rate, respiration) increases in order to deliver enough oxygen to the body's cells. Luckily, the body usually adjusts to high altitudes within a few days, and metabolism returns to normal. Also, be careful when using your blood glucose meter at very high altitudes. Some meters do not give accurate readings above ten thousand feet (check your owner's manual or call the meter manufacturer to see if your meter may be affected).

The Adjustment: Be prepared to lower your basal insulin by 20 to 40 percent for the first couple of days when traveling to high altitudes. This will keep your blood sugar from dropping between meals and while you sleep. Exercising at high altitudes may require a greater dosage reduction than you are used to, as the body has to work extra hard to supply enough oxygen to your muscles.

Nausea

Any time your stomach is upset after eating and bolusing for a meal, you are going to be susceptible to hypoglycemia. When food sits (undigested) in your stomach or is later vomited, you will have taken bolus insulin for something that never actually reached your bloodstream.

The Adjustment: If nausea is common or predictable (such as during early stages of pregnancy or chemotherapy), consider taking your bolus an hour or two *after* eating, once you are certain that your food will stay down.

Otherwise, if your blood sugar is dropping and you are unable to tolerate ordinary food or beverages, there are a few ways to keep your blood sugar from bottoming out. First, try placing glucose tablets or dextrose-containing candy under your tongue or in your cheek. Even without swallowing, some of the sugar can be absorbed through the lining of the mouth. The stomach can sometimes tolerate low-sugar (but not sugar-free) beverages, such as sports drinks or diluted juice, when it cannot tolerate ordinary foods/drinks. Other options include turning the basal rate on your pump down by 80 to 90 percent for a few hours or giving yourself a small injection of glucagon, using an insulin syringe to inject it just below the skin. Ten to twenty units of glucagon are usually sufficient to reverse a downward trend in the blood sugar.

Other Medications

Certain medications, including MAO inhibitors, nicotine patches, antidepressants, and some antibacterial agents, may result in a temporary reduction in blood sugar levels. Starting an oral diabetes medication such as metformin can produce an ongoing need for less insulin, as the liver begins to secrete less than the usual amount of glucose throughout the day and night. The incretin mimetics—Symlin (pramlintide), Byetta (exenatide), and Victoza (liraglutide)—can have a blood sugar–lowering effect by suppressing the pancreas's normal secretion of glucagon.

The Adjustment: Speak to the physician who prescribed the medication to determine whether the dosage warrants any up-front changes in your insulin doses. Otherwise, take a wait-and-see approach. If you notice lower than usual blood sugar levels around the clock after starting (or increasing the dose of) the medication, cut back on your basal insulin in 10 percent increments until the problem is resolved. If the lower readings take place at a consistent time of day, reduce your bolus insulin prior to that time. For example, if you have been going low in the afternoon since starting on a nicotine patch, reduce your lunchtime bolus.

Stuff That Can Make Your
Blood Sugar Rise *or* Fall . . . *or Both*

Just when you think you have it all figured out, along comes a factor or event that can cause blood sugars to both rise and fall, or vice versa. But don't freak out—we can handle these.

Alcohol

Alcoholic beverages that contain carbohydrates, such as beer, table/dessert wine, wine coolers, hard lemonade, frozen/mixed drinks, will raise the blood sugar in the short term. Beer, in fact, is like liquid bread: It raises blood sugar pretty quickly. However, *alcohol* has a tendency to lower blood sugar levels several hours later by keeping the liver from secreting its normal amount of glucose into the bloodstream. As a result, hypoglycemia can occur after drinking. The fact that intoxication often masks the symptoms of hypoglycemia makes the problem worse. Neither the person with diabetes nor people around him/her are aware of the low blood sugar because the hypoglycemic symptoms take on the look, sound, and feel of being drunk. Consequently, preventing hypoglycemia is of paramount importance when drinking.

The Adjustment: When drinking, you should bolus to cover the carbohydrates in your beverages. However, you need to make adjustments to prevent a delayed blood sugar drop from the alcohol. If you use an insulin pump, a temporary basal reduction of 30 to 50 percent for two hours *per drink* can work quite well because on average each alcoholic beverage needs about two hours for the liver to process it (the bigger you are, the less time it takes; the smaller you are, the longer it takes). In other words, if you have three drinks, lower the basal for six hours. Five drinks? Ten hours.

If you take NPH at bedtime, consider lowering the dose by 10 percent for each drink you had that evening, up to an 80 percent reduction. If you take glargine or detemir, take the usual dose but have a modest snack (without bolusing) before going to bed. Ideally, the snack should be of the low-glycemic-index variety so as to provide a steady flow of sugar into the bloodstream for several hours. Examples include nuts, yogurt, chocolate, or carrots.

Impaired Digestion

Gastroparesis is a form of diabetic neuropathy in which the stomach is slow to empty into the intestines. Food digests much slower than usual, so the blood sugar has a tendency to rise several hours after eating rather than right after the meal. Those who take rapid-acting insulin to cover the meals sometimes see a drop in the blood sugar soon after eating, as the insulin begins working but the food doesn't, followed by a sharp rise, as the food kicks in and the insulin wears off.

The Adjustment: You can treat gastroparesis in a variety of ways. Facilitating the movement of food into the intestines is possible with oral medications, electrical stimulation, or modifications to the diet. If these prove to be ineffective, you will need to make mealtime insulin adjustments. Switching from rapid-acting insulin to regular insulin works for many people. Regular's delayed peak (two to three hours after injection) and prolonged action (five to six hours) helps to match the absorption of sugars into the bloodstream for those with slow digestion. Another option is to delay the mealtime bolus until thirty or sixty minutes after the meal. Those who use insulin pumps can extend their bolus over a couple of hours to delay/blunt the peak and prolong the action curve of the insulin.

Menstruation

During various phases of the menstrual cycle, the body produces hormones that can raise or lower blood sugar levels. Many women find that their blood sugar levels are significantly higher for several days before the onset of their period and then lower for a day or two after menses begins. Although the effects of menstrual hormones last around the clock, morning blood sugars seem to be affected the most.

The Adjustment: Note the onset of your period in your self-monitoring records for at least three months. Look for a pattern of consistently high or low blood sugars surrounding your menstrual cycle. Another way to detect this type of pattern is to download your blood glucose meter(s) to the computer and print out a long-term (two- to three-month) trend graph.

In the figure below, menses that began at the end of January produced elevated glucose levels for several days prior (1/26 through 1/29).

Figure 8-3. Trend graph showing a blood glucose rise prior to menses

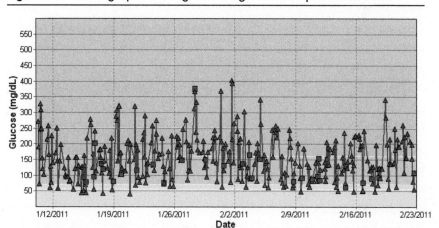

The Adjustment: If you find that you are waking up with high readings before your period begins, take your basal insulin dose up: As soon as premenstrual symptoms appear, raise the nighttime NPH or glargine/levemir dose by 10 to 20 percent or set a temp basal increase of 40 to 50 percent overnight if you use a pump. If your blood sugars run high around the clock prior to your period, raise the basal on your pump for twenty-four hours at a time, or set a secondary basal pattern that you can switch to at the start of your premenstrual phase.

If your blood sugar drops low for the first twenty-four hours after your period begins, reduce your basal insulin dose or cut back on your meal boluses by 20 to 30 percent.

Travel

Travel can present special challenges for people with diabetes. Due to changes in meals, activity, and schedules, blood sugars may vary quite a bit when you travel. Time zone changes can wreak havoc on control because your normal basal insulin patterns may not match your sleep/wake schedule at your destination. When in transit, your blood sugar levels may run higher than usual. This is caused by a combination of factors, including the stress of travel, consumption of restaurant meals, and the fact that prolonged sitting tends to diminish sensitivity to insulin. However, the pattern can change dramatically when you arrive at a vacation destination. The sudden decrease in stress, extra walking, new surroundings to absorb mentally, and (perhaps) warmer temperatures can lead to an overall drop in blood sugar levels.

The Adjustment: Plan to take a little extra basal insulin on travel days but a little less once you arrive and settle in at your destination. Incidentally, if you need to take an insulin injection on a plane using vials and syringes, only inject half as much air as usual into the vial. Cabin pressure is a bit lower than the air pressure on the ground, so you won't need to build up as much pressure inside the vial.

When traveling across time zones, you may need to make some insulin program adjustments. If you use an insulin pump, simply adjust the clock on the pump to correspond with the local time once you arrive. This will help ensure that the peaks and valleys in your basal insulin program will correspond to your sleep schedule at your destination.

Those taking glargine, levemir, or NPH should continue to take the injections twenty-four hours apart. This may mean changing the time of your injection. For example, if you normally take your glargine at 10 p.m. and travel west across three time zones, you should begin taking it at 7 p.m. (local time) once at your destination. Upon traveling home, you can resume your usual injection time of 10 p.m.

Be aware that insulin outside the United States could have a different concentration than the U-100 insulin you are used to using. U-40 insulin is common in some countries, which means that the insulin is only 40 percent as potent as U-100 insulin. If you run out of your insulin and are forced to use U-40 insulin, multiply your usual dose by 2.5. In other words, if you usually take 10 units of U-100 insulin, you will need 25 units of U-40 to get the same effect. If using a pump with U-40 insulin, increase your bolus doses and your basal rates by 250 percent (multiply your usual doses by 2.5).

And remember, insulin is stable at room temperature for up to a month. There is not usually a need to refrigerate your insulin while traveling. However, if the temperature at your destination is in excess of 90 degrees Fahrenheit and your accommodations are not air conditioned, either store your insulin in a refrigerator or bring along a temperature-controlled case for your insulin vials and pens. (See Chapter 10 for travel case options.)

Irregular Sleep

Sleeping isn't just something we do to pass the time at night and during afternoon history classes. Sleep is also a powerful regulator of appetite, energy use, and weight. Lack of sleep can cause an increase in stress hormone production and may cause a rise in blood sugar levels. It also tends to increase appetite and can lead to insulin resistance and weight gain, particularly when normal sleep hours are spent in a sedentary state (watching TV, etc). Conversely, if normal sleep hours are spent working or engaging in physical activity, blood sugars can run lower than usual.

The Adjustment: Be prepared to increase your basal and bolus insulin doses if you are having difficulty sleeping—particularly if you are sleeping less than six hours per night. However, if you are forced (or choose) to work late into the night, you may need to reduce basal insulin temporarily by 20 to 40 percent or have periodic snacks to prevent hypoglycemia.

Just about everyone benefits from maintaining a fairly consistent sleep/wake schedule. If you are having difficulty maintaining a normal sleep pattern, you may benefit from avoiding caffeine, naps, and nighttime exercise (although daytime exercise can be beneficial). Having a comfortable sleep area that you only use for sleeping and engaging in a relaxing activity thirty minutes prior to bedtime are also helpful. In some cases, you can attribute sleep disturbances to emotional upset or an underlying illness. If this is the case, your physician may be able to prescribe appropriate medication or refer you for counseling.

Menopause

Natural menopause is caused by the ovaries progressively reducing estrogen production. Surgical menopause occurs when the ovaries are removed, resulting in a sudden decrease in estrogen. Weight gain often accompanies menopause. Hot flashes, mood swings, and fatigue may occur as levels of estrogen ebb and flow. Because estrogen makes the body more sensitive to insulin, blood sugar control during menopause can become more challenging.

The Adjustment: Many women report more frequent and severe low blood sugars during early menopause, especially during the night. Most find that in the later stages, as estrogen levels decrease permanently, their bodies are more resistant to insulin and that they require higher insulin doses. However, changes in blood sugar levels during menopause are varied and highly individualized. I would hesitate to make permanent changes to your program until a pattern of high or low readings is established over a period of several consecutive days.

Daily fluctuations in estrogen levels are common and can fool you into thinking that you need to make a change in your overall program. Try not to let the seemingly senseless blood sugar variations frustrate you—it is a common and natural occurrence during this phase of your life, but one that should resolve on its own over time.

Symlin (pramlintide)

As presented back in Chapter 3, Symlin is an injectable replacement for the amylin hormone that the beta cells of the pancreas normally secrete (along with insulin). One of Symlin's primary functions is to slow the emptying of the stomach's contents into the small intestine, where the carbs and other nutrients are then absorbed into the bloodstream. When taken along with rapid-acting insulin, Symlin can sometimes cause blood sugar levels to drop soon after eating and then rise a few hours later.

The Adjustment: Although you may not need to alter the *amount* of bolus insulin much (the average bolus reduction is only 10 to 20 percent) when you take Symlin, you will certainly need to alter the *timing*. For those taking injections, I advise you to either take the mealtime rapid-acting insulin after eating or switch to regular insulin. For those using an insulin pump, extending the bolus over one to two hours will provide a better match to the delayed blood sugar rise.

Sports and Exercise

As discussed in the previous chapter, the blood sugar commonly drops during exercise. However, experiencing a blood sugar *rise* at the onset of high-intensity/short-duration exercise and competitive sports is also common. This is caused by a surge of adrenaline that counteracts the effects of insulin and stimulates the liver to release extra sugar into the bloodstream. That's why a two-hour soccer practice can produce much lower blood sugars than a competitive two-hour soccer game—even when the same amount of exercise is performed.

Exercises that often produce a short-term blood sugar rise include:

- weight lifting, particularly when using high weight and low reps;
- sports that involve intermittent bursts of activity, like baseball or golf;
- sprints in events such as running, swimming, rowing, and skating;
- events in which performance is being judged, such as gymnastics or figure skating; and
- sporting events in which winning is the primary objective.

Ironically, the same high-intensity, strenuous sports that produce a short-term blood sugar rise can also produce a delayed blood sugar drop several hours after the activity (as was discussed earlier in this chapter).

The Adjustment: Given that sports performance hinges on having adequate control of one's blood sugar, it is essential that everyone who exercises or competes makes sound adjustments.

I discussed prevention of hypoglycemia through mealtime insulin adjustment in detail in Chapter 7. When you are going to perform aerobic/cardiovascular exercise after a meal, reducing the mealtime rapid-acting insulin is almost always in order.

For Long-Duration Activity

With prolonged exercise (physical activity lasting more than ninety minutes), reducing your basal insulin can be helpful. This is easy to do with an insulin pump: Simply set a temporary basal rate (50 percent of the usual rate is a good place to start) beginning an hour or two before the activity. Setting the temporary basal rate ahead of time ensures that you will have less basal insulin working at the time your activity begins. If you wait until the activity starts to reduce your basal rate, you will have to wait a couple hours to see a noticeable reduction in the level of insulin in your bloodstream. It is important to note that temporary basal reductions (or suspending the pump or disconnecting) are not of much use for preventing lows with activities lasting an hour or less. Basal changes take an hour or two to start having an effect, and the total amount of the insulin being reduced by a temp basal will not be nearly enough to ward off hypoglycemia.

> Temporary basal reductions are not of much use for activities lasting an hour or less.

If you take injections, a reduction in your long-acting insulin dose means that you will be lowering your basal insulin level for nearly twenty-four hours—not just during the time you are exercising. However, this can be useful if your activity is lasting throughout most of the day because you will probably need less basal insulin at night as well. In this case, a 25 percent reduction in your injected basal insulin dose prior to the activity is a good starting point.

With long, intense forms of exercise, preventing hypoglycemia will almost always require a reduction in basal insulin as well as carbohydrate-containing snacks at regular intervals.

Snacking to Prevent Low Blood Sugar

Under certain conditions you will need to eat extra food to prevent hypoglycemia during exercise. For example, when exercise is going to be performed before or between meals, reducing the insulin at the previous meal would only serve to drive the preworkout blood sugar very high. A better approach is to take the normal insulin dose at the previous meal and then snack prior to exercising.

If you decide to exercise soon after you have already taken your usual insulin/medication, snacking will be your only option for preventing hypoglycemia. Also, during very long-duration endurance activities, you may need to eat hourly or half-hourly snacks *in addition* to reducing insulin/medication.

The best *types* of carbohydrates for preventing hypoglycemia during exercise are ones that digest quickly and easily (high-glycemic-index foods). These include sugared beverages (including juices, soft drinks, and sports drinks), bread, crackers, cereal, and low-fat candy.

The size of the snack depends on the duration and intensity of your workout. The harder and longer your muscles are working, the more carbohydrate you will need. The amount is also based on your body size: The bigger you are, the more fuel you will burn while exercising, and thus the more carbohydrate you will need.

Granted, there is no way of knowing *exactly* how much you will need, but the figures in Table 8-2 should serve as a reasonable starting point. To use the chart, line up your approximate body weight with the intensity of the exercise. The grams of carbohydrate represent the amount that you will need prior to *each hour* of activity. If you will be exercising for half an hour, take half the amount indicated. If you will be exercising for two hours, take the full amount at the beginning of each hour. Of course, if your blood sugar is elevated prior to exercising, you will need fewer carbs; if you are below target, you will need additional carbs.

Table 8-2. Carbs to maintain blood sugar during exercise

	Carbohydrate needed (grams) per sixty minutes of physical activity				
	50 lbs (23 kg)	100 lbs (45 kg)	150 lbs (68 kg)	200 lbs (91 kg)	250 lbs (114kg)
Low intensity	5–8g	10–16g	15–25g	20–32g	25–40g
Moderate intensity	10–13g	20–26g	30–40g	40–52g	50–65g
High intensity	15–18g	30–36g	45–55g	60–72g	75–90g

For example, if you weigh 150 pounds (68 kg) and plan a moderate-intensity, forty-five-minute workout, try taking about 25 grams of carb beforehand. If your preworkout blood sugar is elevated, cut back to 10 to 15 grams. If your blood sugar is below target, increase to 35 to 40 grams.

For those who use insulin pumps and choose to lower the basal insulin prior to and during physical activity, the amount of carbohydrate you will need (or the frequency with which you need to eat) will be reduced.

For a more detailed look the carbohydrate required for a variety of different activities, see the "Carb Replacement" chart in Appendix D.

Preventing Blood Sugar Rises During Sports

If you notice that your blood sugar rises during certain types of activities, taking extra insulin beforehand is in your best interest. Case in point: One of my teenage clients always saw his blood sugar drop steadily during hockey practice, though games caused just the opposite effect; his blood sugar would rise well into the 300s (17–22 mmol/l) when he played competitively. When he started taking extra insulin before games, his blood sugar stayed closer to normal, and his speed, stamina, and mental focus all went up a notch. In his first tournament trying this approach, he won his first-ever MVP trophy!

> To prevent a blood sugar rise during sports activity, take a small dose of insulin beforehand.

To determine how much insulin to take before a high-adrenaline form of exercise, consider how much your blood sugar normally rises during the course of an event. If it rises 200 mg/dl (11.2 mmol/l) and your sensitivity factor is 50 (2.8) points per unit, you would normally need to give 4 units of insulin thirty to sixty minutes beforehand. Likewise, if you normally rise 70 mg/dl (3.9 mmol/l) and your sensitivity factor is 30, you will need a little more than 2 units beforehand. However, if you give these full amounts and then start to exercise, you'll probably wind up sucking glucose gel through a straw before too long. My advice is to take *half* of the amount you would usually need to offset the expected blood sugar rise. Likewise, if your blood sugar is elevated prior to an athletic event, give yourself half of your usual correction bolus.

For example, consider our hockey player, Marvin. When Marvin has a game, his blood sugar tends to go up about 150 mg/dl (8.3 mmol/l). His correction factor is 30 mg/dl (1.7 mmol/l) per unit. If his blood sugar before heading for the rink is 200 (11 mmol/l), he needs 2.5 to offset the expected rise (half the 5 units he would normally need) plus 1.5 units to cover his current blood sugar (half the 3 units he would normally take), for a total of 4 units.

If you are nervous about giving insulin before exercise, check your blood sugar more often than usual (perhaps every half hour) and have glucose tablets or some other form of fast-acting carbohydrate nearby. Given the conservative nature of the dosing, your blood sugar is not likely to drop too low. And if it does, fixing a low is much easier than fixing a high during a sport.

Pregnancy

If you have type 1 diabetes, expect your insulin needs to change dramatically through the course of your pregnancy. The proportion of basal (background) to bolus (mealtime) insulin does not change much, but the total amount of insulin required goes through a complete metamorphosis. Do the doses simply rise or fall steadily throughout pregnancy? Of course not! This is *diabetes* we're talking about—nothing is simple.

For most women insulin needs during pregnancy follow a pattern similar to a log flume ride found at an amusement park (see Figure 8-4). Let me explain.

Figure 8-4. Typical insulin requirements through pregnancy

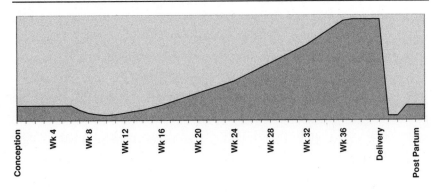

Weeks zero to six: Business as usual. You're just waiting in line to get on the log flume ride, totally oblivious to what you're in for. You probably don't even know you're pregnant, and insulin needs are no different than what they were before you conceived.

Weeks six to twelve: The slight dip. In log flume terms, this is like when you first get into the log boat and the added weight makes it sink slightly into the water. This is truly an amazing phase: You've just found out that you're pregnant, and you're quite excited. As the embryo evolves into a fetus, the autoimmune process that has been destroying your beta cells all these years starts to ease up. This allows your pancreas to start secreting some insulin on its own. The result: a reduction in the need for exogenous (pumped or injected) insulin. Low blood sugar is common during this phase, as many women are taken by surprise that they are producing some of their own insulin again. Severe hypoglycemia is three times more common during the first trimester of pregnancy than during the four months preceding pregnancy.

Weeks twelve to thirty-six: The steady climb. This is the part of the log flume ride when you get on that long, slow conveyer belt up to the top.

You know what happens to your body and the baby during this phase: growth, growth, and more growth. Well, the same thing happens to your insulin needs, despite the fact that your pancreas continues to produce small amounts of insulin. This is due to the increase in your body size as well as the hormones the placenta is producing (including human placental lactogen, progesterone, prolactin, and cortisol), which cause insulin resistance. Total daily insulin needs commonly double or triple during the second and third trimesters of pregnancy.

Weeks thirty-six to delivery: The moment of calm. Once the conveyer belt has brought you to the top, there is always that relaxing, scenic ride before the big plunge. For a few weeks prior to delivery, insulin requirements level off. Things are in a steady state as you make your last-minute preparations.

Delivery: The big plunge. This is what made the log flume famous. Whether your delivery is vaginal or via c-section, insulin needs come down quickly. If you deliver naturally, labor involves a great deal of . . . well . . . labor. And that means reduced insulin needs, as if you were running or lifting weights. And with any form of delivery, the removal of the placenta means a sharp drop-off in hormones that were causing insulin resistance.

One to two days postpartum: The splash. When that log boat comes careening down, it doesn't ease comfortably into the pool of water at the bottom; rather, it torpedoes into it with full force, soaking you and any unfortunate onlookers. Insulin needs do the same thing after delivery: They may actually drop below where they were at the beginning. Remember during the slight-dip phase when we discussed how the pancreas is capable of secreting some insulin on its own? Well, that process continues until shortly after delivery. And when you combine a pancreas that is producing insulin with the sudden elimination of placental hormones along with a sudden decrease in your weight, the results can be astonishing. For the first twenty-four to forty-eight hours postpartum, don't be surprised if insulin needs are dramatically reduced. A small percentage of women don't need to take *any* insulin during this phase!

Home again. It was a wild and crazy ride, but well worth it. Just as the log boat makes its way back to the starting point, insulin needs also tend to find their way back to prepregnancy levels. That's not to say that there won't be any special adjustments necessary. Nursing usually causes the blood sugar to drop modestly. Retained weight will increase insulin needs. And new sleep patterns may require changes to basal insulin levels (as described above).

The Adjustment: During weeks six through ten, reductions to both basal and bolus insulin are usually necessary to prevent frequent bouts of hypoglycemia. A 25 percent reduction in insulin requirements is not uncommon.

During weeks ten through thirty-six, you will need to make steady, gradual increases to both basal and bolus insulin in order to keep up with the increased needs. It is not unusual to see total insulin needs double or triple from preconception until near the end of the third trimester. For the last couple weeks before delivery, insulin needs tend to level off.

During delivery, due to the physical work being performed, women usually need to reduce their basal and bolus insulin doses by approximately 50 percent. Elevated blood sugar during delivery can cause oversecretion of insulin and hypoglycemia in your newborn, so you should cover any highs with rapid-acting insulin, using 50 percent of the usual correction doses, due to the impact of physical labor.

The circle of life. Immediately after delivery insulin doses tend to return to prepregnancy levels. However, if any low blood sugars occur, don't hesitate to make additional reductions for a couple days. Nursing (or pumping breast milk) often requires a small snack to prevent a blood sugar drop. I usually recommend 3 to 5 grams of carb per nursing session during the first couple months, and 5 to 10 grams thereafter.

Chapter Highlights _____

- Secondary factors that tend to raise blood sugar include:
  - anxiety/stress
  - caffeine
  - disease progression
  - protein (in the absence of carbs)
  - large amounts of dietary fat
  - growth and weight gain
  - illness/infection
  - reduced physical activity
  - rebounds from lows
  - steroid medications
  - surgery
- Secondary factors that tend to lower blood sugar include:
  - previous heavy exercise
  - advanced age
  - weight loss
  - heavy brain work
  - heat and humidity
  - nausea
  - high altitude
- Factors that can both raise and lower blood sugar include:
  - alcohol
  - travel
  - intense exercise
  - gastroparesis
  - irregular sleep
  - symlin (pramlintide)
  - menstrual cycles
  - menopause
  - pregnancy

Going to Extremes

"Darling, I don't know why I go to extremes.
Too high or too low, there ain't no in-betweens."

—Billy Joel

Up to this point, I have focused all attention on matching insulin to our precise needs (thinking like a pancreas!). But let's be realistic: With so many variables and factors influencing blood sugar levels, you are going to experience your share of both high and low readings. Even the best-managed people with diabetes have readings that are out of range up to 25 percent of the time.

In this chapter we will focus on what happens when the insulin we take is *not* matched precisely to our body's needs. When we take too much insulin, low blood sugar (hypoglycemia) can occur. Mild forms of hypoglycemia are easily self-treated with a reduction in mealtime insulin or a rapidly digesting snack. However, severe forms of hypoglycemia usually require outside assistance and may lead to loss of consciousness, seizures, coma, or even death.

When we take too little insulin, high blood sugar (hyperglycemia) occurs. We can treat most garden-variety episodes of hyperglycemia with correction insulin. However, a severe lack of insulin in the body can result in a life-threatening condition known as diabetic ketoacidosis (DKA). Because death is something we generally try to avoid, I will present strategies for both preventing and treating severe hypoglycemia and DKA in this chapter. I'll also take a close look at ways to prevent after-meal highs, commonly referred to as "spikes."

The Science Behind Hypoglycemia

Hypoglycemia (hereafter referred to as a "low") is the main limiting factor in intensive diabetes management. Without the risk of lows we could simply load up on insulin and never have another high reading. Or, as my wife so eloquently reminds me from time to time, "Any idiot can have a decent A1c if they're taking too much insulin and going low all the time!"

Low blood sugar affects virtually all systems of the body, but none quite as much as the brain. Brain cells are picky about their fuel source: They only like to burn sugar for energy. Brain and nerve cells have another special feature: They do not require insulin to absorb sugar. Instead, they have special built-in transporters that shuttle sugar across the cell membrane without the aid of insulin.

Low blood sugar is usually defined as a level of less than 70 mg/dl (3.9 mmol/l). Mild lows can cause inconvenience, embarrassment, poor physical and mental performance, impaired judgment, mood changes, weight gain, and rebound high blood sugars. Severe lows can induce seizures, loss of consciousness, coma, or even death. Repeated or prolonged bouts of severe hypoglycemia have the potential to cause permanent mental impairment, although this is usually seen only in the most extreme cases.

Mild Lows

Soon after diabetes is diagnosed, the central nervous system detects hypoglycemia quickly and easily. In some cases, symptoms can occur even at blood sugars above 70 (3.9). Blood sugars in the 80s or 90s

(4s–5s), or a rapid drop from a very high level toward a more normal level, may induce hypoglycemic symptoms.

Upon sensing that the blood sugar is low, the brain sends a signal to the adrenal gland, which releases a surge of adrenaline. Adrenaline, in turn, stimulates the liver to secrete extra sugar into the bloodstream and partially blocks the action of insulin. Adrenaline also causes a number of physical symptoms: rapid heartbeat, perspiration, shaking, hunger, and a generally anxious feeling. (You may recognize these as the same symptoms that occur when you are under intense stress, like when your mother-in-law calls to tell you she's coming to move in.) At this point most people are capable of thinking rationally and consuming food in order to raise their blood sugar level.

Moderate Lows

If blood sugar levels are allowed to drop into the 50s or 40s (3–2 mmol/l), the brain begins losing the ability to function. Confusion usually sets in, accompanied by dizziness and weakness. Speech may become slurred. You may exhibit unusual emotions such as irritability or despair. Vision may become blurred. You will have a difficult time thinking clearly and co-ordinating your movements. At this point you may or may not be able to think rationally enough to consume food to raise your blood sugar. In many instances a friend or family member will need to assist you.

Severe Lows

An extreme or extended blood sugar drop may cause you to pass out or experience a seizure. Very severe, prolonged lows can result in coma or death. Severe lows, by definition, require outside assistance and are usually treated with an injection of glucagon or an intravenous infusion of dextrose.

The DEVOlution of Symptoms

No, it's not a typo. And it has nothing to do with the band Devo ("Whip It," circa 1980). The symptoms of hypoglycemia do not evolve: They devolve, or break down, over time. The brain becomes more efficient at extracting glucose from the bloodstream after going years with off-and-on low blood sugars. In other words, the brain will cease to detect mild low blood sugars; it produces little or no adrenaline response, and physical symptoms (shaking, sweating, etc.) fail to take place. Thus, there may be no warning of low blood sugar in its early stages. The first symptoms are those of a moderate low blood sugar (confusion, etc.), and these may not occur until the blood sugar is already at a dangerously low level.

The name given to this phenomenon is "hypoglycemia unawareness." It affects most people who have had diabetes for several years and tends to become worse over time. The more lows you have, the less likely you are to experience any warning signs the next time. Quite a paradox!

Research has shown that the early symptoms of low blood sugar can, to some extent, be restored by avoiding lows over an extended period of time. People with severe cases of hypoglycemia unawareness have been able to reestablish their early warning symptoms by going several weeks without any readings below 80 (4.4). Although this process may require a temporary increase in the HbA1c level, it is well worth it to be able to detect lows and prevent severe hypoglycemia.

Treatment of Lows

Diabetes is a tricky disease. Low blood sugars sometimes feel like highs, and highs sometimes feel like lows. If you suspect that your blood sugar is low, take a few seconds to confirm it by checking your blood sugar. I can't tell you how many times I thought I was low, only to test and get a reading in the 200s or 300s (teens to 20s). High blood sugars can cause symptoms similar to those caused by lows (tiredness, hunger, a jittery feeling). Getting an exact reading will also help to determine how much carb you need to treat the low.

With premeal blood sugars that are below your target but above 70 mg/dl (3.9 mmol/l), reducing your meal bolus using your correction formula is a sound approach. For readings below 70, you should treat the low immediately, wait ten to fifteen minutes for the blood sugar to come up, and then have your meal (giving the usual dose for your meal). If you feed the low *and* reduce your mealtime bolus, you will have double treated and will probably wind up quite high.

> There is no one-size-fits-all when it comes to treating lows.

There is no one-size-fits-all treatment for hypoglycemia. Proper treatment depends on a number of factors, including:

1. *Body size:* The bigger you are, the more carbs you will need to raise your blood sugar. If you weigh less than 60 pounds (28 kg), each gram of carbohydrate should raise your blood sugar about 6 to 10 mg/dl (0.33–0.55 mmol/l); if you weigh 60 to 100 pounds (29–47 kg), each gram should raise you about 5 mg/dl (0.28); at 101 to 160 pounds (48–76 kg), the rise is about 4 points (0.22); 161 to 220 pounds (77–105 kg), about 3 points (0.17); over 220 pounds (105 kg), 2 points (0.11).

2. *Blood sugar level:* The lower your blood sugar, the more carbs you will need to get back up to normal. Table 9-1 provides a good starting point. The goal on this chart is to raise the blood sugar to about 120 mg/dl (6.7 mmol/l). If your specific blood sugar target is more or less than 120, you will need more or fewer carbs than the amount listed.

Table 9-1. Proper treatment for low blood sugar (based on body weight and blood sugar level)

Carbs needed to raise blood sugar to approximately 120 mg/dl (6.7 mmol/l):					
Blood Sugar	60s (3.3–3.9)	50s (2.8–3.2)	40s (2.2–2.7)	30s (1.7–2.1)	20s (1.1–1.6)
Weight:					
<60 lbs (28 kg)	9g	11g	13g	15g	17g
60–100 lbs (29–47 kg)	11g	13g	15g	17g	19g
101–160 lbs (48–76 kg)	14g	16g	19g	21g	24g
161–220 lbs (77–105 kg)	18g	22g	25g	28g	32g
>220 (>105 kg)	28g	33g	38g	43g	48g

3. *The rate of change:* This is easily seen on a continuous glucose monitor. If your blood sugar is low and still dropping quickly, you will need
more carb than the standard amount. (See Figure 9-1.) If you are low
and leveling off, the standard amount should work fine. (See Figure 9-2.)
Rapid blood sugar drops are most common when you are still in the peak
phase of your mealtime bolus insulin, in the midst of exercising.

Figure 9-1. Blood glucose low and   **Figure 9-2.** Blood glucose low but
accelerating downward   leveling off

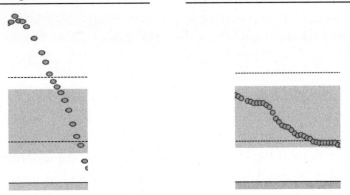

The following formula can be used to determine your precise carb
needs:

$$\text{grams of carb needed to treat a low} =$$
$$(\text{target BG} - \text{actual BG}) / \text{rise per gram of carb}$$

For example, if your target is 100, your blood sugar is 62, and each
gram of carb raises you 3 points, you will need (100–62) / 3, or 13 grams
of carb.

Remember, all carbs are not created equal. Some will raise your
blood sugar very quickly, whereas others will take their sweet time
(excuse the play on words). When your blood sugar is low, choose a
food that will raise you as quickly as possible. Refer to the glycemic index and select foods with a score of at least 70. Examples of high-
glycemic-index foods that are portable and measurable include:

dextrose* (GI =102)
dry cereal (70–90)
pretzels (81)
jelly beans (80)
gatorade (78)
vanilla wafers (77)
graham crackers (74)
plain bread/crackers (70–75)
LifeSavers (70)

*Dextrose-containing foods include glucose tablets/gels, SweeTarts, Smarties, Spree, AirHeads, Runts, Nerds, and BottleCaps.

Foods with a lower glycemic index, such as whole fruit, milk, ice cream, and—hate to say it—chocolate, are not the best choices for treating lows. They will take significantly longer to raise your blood sugar. Many people overtreat their lows by continuing to eat until the symptoms disappear. It usually takes ten to fifteen minutes for high glycemic index foods to raise the blood sugar, and twenty to sixty minutes for low glycemic index foods. Be patient! If you suspect that your blood sugar has not come up enough, test it to find out. If your blood sugar is still below 70 (3.9) fifteen minutes after treatment, go ahead and eat a little bit more.

If you happen to go overboard on the treatment of your low (as we all do on occasion), cover the excess carbs with insulin. For example, if you normally take 1 unit for every 10 grams of carb and you overtreat your low by 40 grams, give yourself 4 units of insulin once your blood sugar has risen back to normal. Otherwise, your blood sugar will rise well above your target in the next couple of hours.

Treating Severe Lows

You must treat severe hypoglycemia (when a person is unwilling or unable to consciously swallow food) differently than you would mild and moderate lows. Putting any kind of food into the mouth of someone having a severe low is dangerous. They could choke on the food and suffocate, or they could instinctively bite down and take the fingers off the person trying to feed them.

There are two things—and only two things—you should do to treat someone having a severe low blood sugar: Call for emergency help and administer an injection of glucagon (or Glucagen).

Glucagon (or brand name Glucagen) is a hormone (like insulin) that raises blood sugar by stimulating the liver to release its stored-up sugar into the bloodstream. It will usually work in ten to twenty minutes. Glucagon is a prescription item that comes in a kit containing a large, fluid-filled syringe, a small vial with the glucagon hormone in powder form, and instructions written in a seemingly foreign language. The kits have an expiration date (they are usually good for about eighteen months), so check them periodically to make sure yours is fresh. If possible, save your expired kits and allow your partner to practice with them (on a pillow or foam ball—not you!).

There are several steps involved in administering glucagon, and it may be difficult to perform them exactly right in a highly stressful situation. But it is certainly worth the effort. The good news is that work is under way to develop glucagon in a premixed formulation (no mixing necessary!), so all you would need to do is take the syringe out of the case and inject. The procedure for administering glucagon, in *plain English*, is as follows:

1. Call 911. Have paramedics on the way in case the glucagon injection fails to work.
2. Pull the cap off the syringe and flip the cap off the vial.
3. Inject all of the fluid into the vial.
4. Remove the syringe from the vial. Keep pressure on the plunger to make sure air does not escape from the vial.
5. Shake or swirl the vial gently until the fluid is evenly mixed (no clumps) and mostly clear.
6. With the vial held upside down, reinsert the tip of the needle into the vial. (Do *not* put the whole needle in; you will draw in air accidentally!)

7. Draw the fluid into the syringe. For very small children (under age six), draw in ⅓ cc; for children six to twelve, draw in ½ cc; over age twelve, draw in 1 cc.

8. Insert the needle straight (not at an angle) into a muscle such as the thigh, buttocks, or shoulder. Inject the full contents of the syringe.

9. Remove the syringe and apply a tissue to suppress any bleeding.

10. Turn the victim onto his or her side to prevent choking (in case vomiting occurs).

The victim should regain consciousness in ten to twenty minutes. If he or she does not, wait for paramedics to arrive. Contact your health care team to troubleshoot and work on a plan for preventing the severe low from happening again.

Note: Everyone who takes insulin is at risk for severe hypoglycemia. It is important to wear medical identification at all times. The Medic Alert Foundation provides more than just medical I.D. jewelry: It maintains a database of medical information that paramedics will have instant access to when they call in. Bracelets and necklaces are recommended because these are the first things paramedics will look for when they arrive at the scene.

Preventing Lows

Minimizing the incidence of low blood sugar can go a long way toward protecting your personal safety and keeping blood sugar levels from bouncing around too much as a result of rebounds. Minimizing the incidence of lows is also the best way to ensure that you will experience early symptoms when your blood sugar is dropping and thus be able to treat the low before it becomes severe.

Experiencing a couple of mild low blood sugars per week is usually acceptable. However, if they are occurring more often or if they are of a severe nature, try applying these strategies:

Match Your Insulin to Your Needs

The first step in preventing lows is the same as the first step in achieving tight control: Mimic the action of a healthy pancreas as closely as possible. Daytime doses of NPH in particular do not match the basal/bolus insulin secretion of the pancreas nearly as well as programs that utilize basal insulin. NPH insulin can peak at inconsistent and inappropriate times, thereby increasing the odds of low blood sugar. Switching to a true basal insulin (glargine, detemir, or an insulin pump) will greatly reduce your risk for hypoglycemia.

Use Rapid-Acting Insulin

Rapid-acting insulin analogs (Humalog, Novolog/NovoRapid, Apidra) tend to produce fewer low blood sugars than regular insulin does. Their rapid onset, consistent peak, and short duration of action match up well to the absorption of carbohydrates in most meals. Regular insulin peaks later and lasts significantly longer. It has a tendency to make blood sugars drop three to six hours after eating—long after the food has been digested and absorbed into the bloodstream.

Dose Properly

Accidental overdosing of insulin is a common cause of hypoglycemia. If you are on relatively low doses (less than 5 units per injection), look for syringes or pens that offer half-unit markings so that you can dose more precisely. You also have the option of diluting your insulin for more precise dosing, as I described in Chapter 4. If you have difficulty seeing your syringes, use an insulin pen or injection aid. (See Chapter 10.) If necessary, have someone else draw up your syringes. And *pay attention to your math!* A single incorrect calculation can send your blood sugar spiraling downward. If you accidentally take too much insulin, drink or eat enough carbs to offset the extra dose and then check your blood sugar hourly until the insulin wears off.

Give Your Insulin Time to Work

As discussed in Chapter 7, boluses of rapid-acting insulin do not stop working after just an hour or two; rather, they typically take three to five hours to finish working. When figuring the amount of correction insulin needed to bring a high blood sugar down to normal, taking the unused portion of your previous boluses into account is important. Likewise, figuring the amount of bolus insulin required to cover a meal should be based on the blood sugar three to four hours after the meal. If you set your doses so that your blood sugar is down to normal two hours after eating, you are likely to experience hypoglycemia within the next couple of hours.

Time Your Boluses Properly

Foods that have a low glycemic index value tend to take a while to raise the blood sugar level. Very large meals that contain a great deal of fat can also take a while to raise the blood sugar. Giving a bolus before or during these types of meals can cause low blood sugar soon after eating. Instead, plan to give your boluses after eating or, if using an insulin pump, program the bolus to be delivered over an extended period of time. These strategies are also helpful for preventing post-meal blood sugar drops when using Symlin (pramlintide), Byetta (exenatide), or Victoza (liraglutide).

Set Appropriate Targets

The lower your target blood sugar, the greater your chances for hypoglycemia—plain and simple. Target blood sugars of 80 or 90 (4.4–5.0) leave little margin for error. Even the slightest bit of extra exercise or a minor overestimate of carbohydrates will probably result in a low. A target of 100 (5.6) or more allows a bit more breathing room. Some people change their target BG from day to day based on their risk for lows. If you're coming off a day when a low occurred, your BG was very erratic, or you exercised heavily, your risk for hypoglycemia is increased. Raising your target modestly can save you from lows.

Also, make sure your correction formulas are set properly. A sensitivity factor that is set too low will cause overdosing for high readings and lead to hypoglycemia. As mentioned in Chapter 7, sensitivity factors are often higher at night than they are during the day. And don't forget to *reduce* your mealtime boluses any time the blood sugar is below target.

Time Meals and Snacks Appropriately

When using any type of intermediate- or long-acting insulin, consuming your meals and snacks on a consistent schedule is imperative. A delay of as little as half an hour (when using daytime NPH) or an hour (when using glargine or detemir) can cause a significant drop in blood sugar. If you anticipate a meal delay, consume part of your usual meal in the form of a carbohydrate-containing snack.

Discount Fiber Grams

Don't forget: Fiber is included in the "total carbohydrate" listings on food labels, but it does not raise blood sugar levels. Any time you are consuming a food item that contains fiber, subtract it from the total carbohydrate before calculating your meal bolus.

Adjust for Exercise and Daily Activity

Physical activity of almost any kind (from running laps to running a vacuum) will accelerate muscle cells' uptake of glucose. In those without diabetes insulin secretion comes to a grinding halt and production of counter-regulatory hormones increases at the onset of exercise. This helps to maintain blood sugars within normal limits. For those who take insulin, however, adjustments must be made to prevent low blood sugar during and after exercise. For activity performed after a meal, you will probably need to reduce the meal bolus. Activity before or between meals will probably require an extra snack. Prolonged or very strenuous activity may require reductions in both basal and bolus insulin, along with periodic snacks. Following exhaustive forms of exercise, you should make adjustments to prevent a delayed blood sugar drop.

Adjust for Alcohol

In Chapter 8 we discussed how alcohol can cause a delayed drop in blood sugar by suppressing the liver's secretion of glucose. After drinking be sure to either lower your basal insulin level for several hours or consume extra snacks to compensate.

Check, Check, Check

Very few of us are good at guessing our blood sugar levels with much precision, especially when the readings are not particularly high or low. Frequent blood sugar checks will allow you to catch many below-target readings before they turn into hypoglycemia. For instance, a bedtime reading of 82 (4.6) may seem innocuous, but even a slight drop during the night would result in a low blood sugar. Knowing that the reading is close to low allows you the opportunity to have a small snack, thus reducing the likelihood of hypoglycemia during the night.

Use a Continuous Glucose Monitor

> CGMs allow us to prevent low blood sugar and catch them as early as possible.

Continuous glucose monitors provide the user with low blood sugar alerts. The threshold for the alert can be set above the level at which you begin to notice symptoms so that you can catch your lows as early as possible. Some CGM systems also provide *predictive* alerts: If they anticipate that you will go low based on the current glucose level and direction the blood sugar is headed, it can alert you. Others provide *rate of change* alerts, which can let you know if your blood sugar is drop-ping very quickly—even if it is still in a normal range—so that you can decide whether you need a snack to prevent hypoglycemia.

Overall, continuous glucose monitors are effective tools for reduc-ing the incidence of low blood sugar and catching them as early as possible. Research has shown that the average length of low blood sugar episodes is cut in half when the low alerts are used. This is very important because the length of a low, and not necessarily the severity of the low, is what puts us at risk for seizures and loss of consciousness.

Dealing with Postmeal Highs

At the opposite end of the spectrum from lows are high blood sugar levels. An almost unlimited number of factors can cause highs, but you can usually prevent (and always fix) them with additional insulin.

One type of high that causes frustration for many people is the one that occurs soon after eating. We call this a "postmeal spike." Post-meal spikes are temporary high blood sugars that occur approximately one to two hours after eating. It is normal for the blood sugar to rise a small amount after eating, even in people who do not have diabetes. However, if the spike is too high, it can affect your quality of life today and contribute to serious health problems down the road.

The reason blood sugar spikes very high after eating for many people with diabetes is a simple matter of timing. In a person without diabetes, consumption of carbohydrate results in two important reactions: the immediate release of insulin into the bloodstream and the production of amylin. Insulin produced by the pancreas starts working almost immedi-ately and finishes its job in a matter of minutes. Amylin keeps food from reaching the intestines too quickly (where the nutrients are absorbed into the bloodstream). As a result, the moment blood sugar starts to rise, insulin is there to sweep the extra sugar into the body's cells. In most cases, the after-meal blood sugar rise is barely noticeable.

> The reason blood sugar spikes after a meal is that insulin is too slow to cover most of the food we eat.

However, people with diabetes are like a baseball player with very slow reflexes. We're in the batter's box facing a pitcher who throws 98-mph fastballs; by the time we swing, the ball is already in the catcher's mitt. Rapid-acting insulin that is injected (or infused by a pump) takes approximately fifteen minutes to start working, sixty to ninety minutes to peak, and three to five hours to finish working. And don't forget about the amylin hormone effect. In people type 2 diabetes, amylin is produced in insufficient amounts. Those with type 1 diabetes produce none at all. As a result, food digests even *faster* than usual. This combination of slower insulin and faster food digestion can cause blood sugar to rise quite high soon after eating. This is followed by a sharp drop once the mealtime insulin finally kicks in.

Why Are Spikes a Problem?

Even though the spike is temporary, all of those spikes throughout the day can raise your HbA1c. Maintaining an A1c below 7 percent without paying attention to after-meal blood sugar levels is difficult. Scientists and doctors have studied the long-term effects of postmeal highs extensively. For those with type 1 diabetes, significant postmeal rises have been shown to produce earlier onset of kidney disease and accelerate the progression of existing eye problems (retinopathy). And postmeal hyperglycemia is an independent risk factor for cardiovascular problems for those with type-2 diabetes.

But the problems are not limited to long-term complications. Any time blood sugars rise particularly high—even temporarily—our quality of life suffers. Energy decreases, brain function falters, physical/athletic abilities become diminished, and moods become altered. During pregnancy even mild rises in blood sugar after meals have been associated with excessive and unhealthy growth of the baby.

Measurement and Goals

The exact timing of blood sugar spikes can vary from person to person and meal to meal. However, on average the postmeal peak tends to occur about one hour and fifteen minutes after starting a meal. So checking your blood sugar (using a fingerstick) about an hour after finishing a meal should provide a good indication of how much of a spike is taking place. Continuous glucose monitors provide trend graphs that make seeing exactly what is happening after meals easy. See the example in Figure 9-3.

Figure 9-3. CGM display showing postmeal peaks

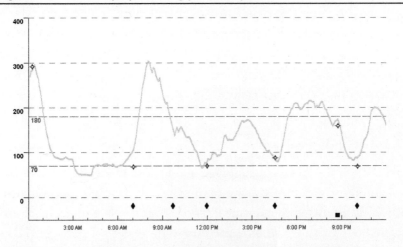

Another way to assess after-meal blood sugar control is through a blood test called "GlycoMark." Just as an HbA1c measures average blood sugar for the past few months, GlycoMark measures the degree to which blood sugars are spiking over the past couple of weeks. Glyco-Mark measures the level of a specific type of sugar that becomes *depleted* whenever the kidneys are spilling sugar into the urine (typically when BG exceeds approximately 180mg/dl or 10 mmol/l). Ask your physician if this test is available to you.

The American Diabetes Association recommends keeping blood sugar below 180 mg/dl (10 mmol/l) one to two hours after eating. The

European Diabetes Policy Group recommends keeping it below 165 mg/dl at the peak, and the American Association of Clinical Endocrinologists and International Diabetes Federation suggest keeping it below 140 mg/dl after eating. However, no specific guidelines are provided for type 1 versus type 2 diabetes, insulin users versus noninsulin users, or children versus adults. (Not surprisingly, none of these groups suggest *how* to meet those goals either.)

A summary of my recommendations for postmeal glucose is listed in Table 9-2.

Table 9-2. Summary of after-meal blood sugar targets

Group/age	Postmeal goal
Adults taking mealtime insulin	<180 mg/dl (10 mmol/l)
Adolescents with type 1	<200 mg/dl (11)
School-age children with type 1	<225 mg/dl (12.5)
Preschool/toddlers with type 1	<250 mg/dl (14)
Women during pregnancy	<140 mg/dl (8)
Type 2s taking basal insulin only	<160 mg/dl (9)

Spike Control

If your doctor's only answer for controlling the after-meal spikes is "Just take more insulin," think again. Increasing the *amount* of insulin does little to reduce the immediate postmeal spike, but it will almost surely make you go low before the next meal.

To reduce the spike, you can use a number of strategies. Some involve medications, whereas others involve daily lifestyle patterns.

1. Choose the right insulin (or medication)

The right insulin or medication program can make or break your ability to control those after-meal spikes. In general, insulin and medications that work quickly and for a short period of time will work better than those that work slowly over a prolonged period of time.

If you are still using regular insulin at mealtimes (or daytime NPH to cover your midday meal), switch to a rapid-acting insulin analog (Humalog, Novolog/NovoRapid, or Apidra). If you have type 2 diabetes and take a sulfonylureas (glyburide, glipizide, glimepiride), switch to a rapid (and shorter)-acting meglitinide (repaglinide, nateglinide). Another class of diabetes medications that can improve after-meal control by partially blocking the transport of sugars across the intestines and into the bloodstream is called "alpha-glucosidase inhibitors." However, be aware that this class of medications can cause gastrointestinal upset, gas, and bloating.

2. Back Up Your Bolus
As I discussed in Chapter 7, the timing of your mealtime insulin can make a huge difference in your postmeal control. Boluses given too late to match the entry of sugars into the bloodstream can produce significant hyperglycemia soon after eating, whereas a properly timed bolus can result in excellent after-meal control. In general, giving your bolus fifteen to twenty minutes before eating should result in less of a spike than bolusing just before or during your meals.

3. Use a Jet Injector
Jet injectors are insulin injection devices that spray insulin through the skin at a high speed in a "mist" form. By spreading the insulin molecules over a wider area under the skin than syringes, pens, and pumps do, the insulin starts working faster, peaks earlier and stronger, and finishes working sooner.

4. Bolus for the Basal
In order to have more insulin working right after eating and less working several hours later, a pump user can run a temporary basal reduction for three hours just before eating and give a normal bolus equal to the basal insulin that would have been delivered. For example, if your basal rate in the morning is .7 units per hour, you could bolus an extra 2 units before breakfast and then set a temp basal of 10 percent (90 percent reduction) for the next three hours.

5. Use an Incretin

Three injectable hormones—Symlin (pramlintide) and Byetta (exenatide) have powerful effects on postmeal blood sugar. Both slow gastric emptying and keep carbohydrates from raising the blood sugar too quickly after meals. They also blunt appetite and inhibit secretion of the blood sugar–raising hormone glucagon after meals. Of the two, Symlin (taken before eating) tends to produce the best aftermeal control.

6. Think Lower GI

As I discussed in Chapter 7, glycemic index (GI) refers to the *speed* with which food raises the blood sugar level. Although all carbohydrates (except for fiber) convert into blood sugar eventually, some carbs do so much faster than others do. As a general rule, switching to lower-GI foods will help reduce your after-meal blood sugar spikes. Table 9-3 shows some examples.

Table 9-3. Substituting low-GI for high-GI foods

Meal	High-GI choices	Lower-GI choices
Breakfast	typical cereal, bagel, toast, waffles, pancakes, corn muffins, juice, breakfast bars	high-fiber cereal, oatmeal, yogurt, whole fruit, milk, bran muffin, granola
Lunch	sandwiches on white bread/rolls, French fries, tortillas, canned pasta, most microwave meals	chili, rye/pumpernickel/sourdough bread, corn, carrots, salad vegetables
Dinner	rice, couscous, rolls, white potato, canned vegetables	sweet potato, pasta, beans, fresh/steamed vegetables
Snacks	pretzels, chips, crackers, cake, cookies	popcorn, fruit, chocolate, ice cream, nuts

7. Add Some Acidity

A food property that directly affects the rate of digestion is acidity. This is why sourdough bread has a much lower GI value than regular bread does. Research has shown that adding acidity in the form of *vinegar* (straight or in dressing/condiment form) can reduce the one-hour post-meal blood sugar rise by as much as 50 percent.

8. Split Your Meal

If you are having a meal and don't want your blood sugar to rise all at once, consider saving a portion of your meal for a snack one or two hours later. Still give the full mealtime insulin before eating any of the meal—just don't eat all of the food right away. For example, if you have a bowl of cereal and juice for breakfast, bolus for the full meal before eating anything. Then have the cereal at breakfast time and postpone the juice until mid-morning.

9. Get Moving

Being physically active after eating can reduce postmeal spikes in a number of ways. The enhanced blood flow helps the insulin absorb and act more quickly. Muscle activity diverts blood flow away from the intestines, resulting in slower absorption of sugars into the bloodstream. Plus, the working muscles consume some of the sugar that enters the bloodstream.

How much activity is required to experience these benefits? Not much. Ten or fifteen minutes (or more) of *mild* activity will usually get the job done. The key is to avoid *sitting* for extended periods of time after eating. Instead of reading, watching TV, or working on the computer, go for a walk, shoot some hoops, or do some chores. Try to schedule your active tasks (housework, yard work, shopping, walking pets) for *after* meals.

10. Prevent Hypoglycemia

Low blood sugar is problematic in many ways. One of the body's responses to hypoglycemia is accelerated gastric emptying: Food digests and raises blood sugar even more rapidly than usual. Although this is certainly a desirable phenomenon (who wants to wait for food to kick in during a low?), when it occurs before meals it will contribute to an excessive postmeal rise. Preventing hypoglycemia prior to meals and snacks is yet another strategy to "strike the spike."

The Other Extreme: Ketoacidosis

DKA (diabetic ketoacidosis) is a condition in which the blood becomes highly acidic as a result of dehydration and excessive ketone (acid) production. When bodily fluids become acidic, some of the body's systems stop functioning properly. It is a serious condition that will make you violently ill and can kill you. The primary cause of DKA is a lack of working insulin in the body. Let me explain.

> The primary cause of DKA is a lack of working insulin.

Normal Fuel Metabolism

Most of the body's cells burn primarily sugar (glucose) for energy. Many cells also burn fat, but in much smaller amounts. Glucose happens to be a very "clean" form of energy—there are virtually no waste products left over when cells burn it up. Fat, however, is a "dirty" source of energy. When fat is burned, the cells produce waste products, which are called "ketones." Ketones are acid molecules that can pollute the bloodstream and affect the body's delicate pH balance if produced in large quantities. Luckily, we don't tend to burn huge amounts of fat at one time, and the ketones that are produced can be broken down during the process of glucose metabolism; glucose and ketones can "jump into the fire" together.

As you can tell, having an ample supply of glucose in the body's cells is important. That requires two things: sugar (glucose) in the bloodstream and insulin to shuttle the sugar into the cells. (See Figure 9-4.)

Figure 9-4. Normal fuel metabolism

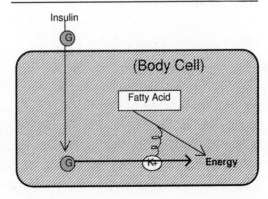

Abnormal Fuel Metabolism

What would happen if you had no insulin? I'm not talking about a minor under-dosage; I'm talking about having none whatsoever. A number of things would start to go wrong. Without insulin glucose cannot get into the body's cells. As a result, the cells begin burning large amounts of fat for energy. This, of course, leads to the production of large amounts of ketones. Although some of the ketones eventually spill over into the urine, the body is unable to eliminate sufficient amounts to restore a healthy pH balance in the bloodstream. (See Figure 9-5.)

Figure 9-5. Fuel metabolism in the absence of insulin

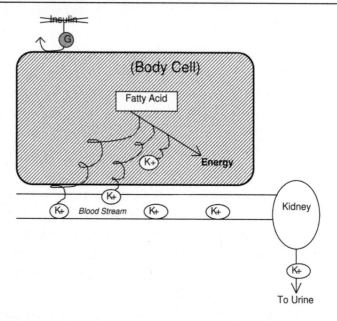

Dehydration further complicates the problem. Without sufficient insulin to inhibit the liver's secretion of sugar, large amounts of glucose are released into the bloodstream. Because high blood sugar causes excessive urination, dehydration ensues. Without glucose metabolism to help break down the ketones and without ample fluids to help neutralize them, the bloodstream and tissues of the body become very acidic. This is a state of ketoacidosis.

Causes and Prevention of Ketoacidosis

What can cause a sudden lack of insulin in the body? There are a number of potential culprits.

Illness, Infection, and Dehydration

Illness, infection, and dehydration can cause the production of large quantities of stress hormones, which counteract insulin. In other words, during an illness, you could have insulin in your body, but it is rendered almost useless because stress hormones are blocking its action.

Prevention: The sick-day strategies presented in Chapter 8 are worth reviewing. During an illness, insulin requirements are usually increased—even if you are not eating as much as usual. Keep taking your basal insulin regardless of your food intake. If your blood sugars are running high or if ketones are present in your urine, you will need to drink lots of water, and you may need to increase your dose of basal insulin by 50 to 100 percent.

Lack of Carbohydrates

A lack of carbohydrates in the diet can also induce ketone production. During periods of starvation, prolonged fasting, or restricted carbohydrate intake, the body's cells must resort to burning alternative sources of fuel, namely fat and protein. With increased fat metabolism and limited carbohydrate metabolism, ketone production may exceed the body's ability to eliminate them.

Prevention: Ketone production is unhealthy for anyone, particularly those with diabetes. Maintaining at least a modest level of carbohydrate intake throughout the day should prevent ketosis. If you must fast for short periods of time, talk with your doctor to ensure that it will not interfere with any other health conditions or medications that you may be taking.

You can usually fast safely by taking only basal insulin, with rapid-acting insulin as touch-ups for high blood sugars. If you take intermediate-acting insulin (NPH) in the morning, take half of your usual dose. Be sure to check your blood sugar level regularly during a fast. If your blood sugar drops below 70 (3.9), you must snack to bring it back up.

Losing Weight When You Take Insulin

There is nothing magical about very-low-carb diets when it comes to weight loss. Research has shown that just about any reasonable diet plan that has you paying close attention to what you are eating will result in weight loss.

Losing weight when you take insulin can be challenging, but there are ways to make it happen. Ultimately, anything that allows you to take *less* insulin while still maintaining your blood sugar control will promote weight loss.

Ways to cut back on basal insulin

- reducing overall stress levels
- minimizing high-fat foods
- increasing daily walking/activity
- increasing muscle mass
- taking metformin

Ways to cut back on bolus insulin

- reducing carb portions
- increasing fiber intake
- postmeal exercise
- reducing snack frequency
- using Symlin, Byetta, or Victoza

If you are working to lose weight and experience more than one low blood sugar per week at the same time of day, cut back on the insulin dose that is working prior to that time. Repeated bouts of hypoglycemia will make it very, very difficult to lose weight. Conversely, cutting insulin back will facilitate weight loss.

Spoiled Insulin

Using spoiled insulin can lead to high blood sugar and ketone production. Insulin that has been frozen or exposed to extreme heat can "denature," or break down so that the insulin molecules no longer work. Using the same vial or cartridge of insulin for many months or using it past its expiration date can also cause problems.

Prevention: You should not use insulin vials and cartridges after their expiration date. Once you begin using a vial or cartridge, discard it after a couple of months (the insulin makers recommend starting new insulin vials/pens monthly). Keep your unopened insulin stored in the refrigerator, in an area that is not likely to freeze, such as the butter compartment. Before using a new insulin vial or cartridge, look for clumps, crystals on the glass, or discoloration. If you suspect that the insulin has gone bad, it probably has. When ordering insulin by mail, ask that it be shipped in a temperature-controlled container. Keep your insulin in your carry-on when you travel, as luggage may be exposed to extreme temperatures.

Poor Absorption

Poor absorption at the injection site can also cause an insulin deficiency. Remember, once insulin is injected or infused under the skin, it must absorb into the bloodstream in order to take effect. If the insulin "pockets" under the skin, it may never work. In some cases, the insulin may absorb much later than expected, resulting in a high blood sugar, followed by an unanticipated low.

Prevention: Just as you rotate your tires to prevent uneven tread wear, you must rotate your injection and infusion (pump) sites to prevent uneven insulin absorption. Injecting the same spots repeatedly can cause lipodystrophy—a breakdown or inflammation of the fat tissue below the skin. When this happens the skin can either dimple or become unusually hard and insensitive. One of my clients calls these "happy spots" because they don't hurt at all when giving a shot or inserting an infusion set. The problem with happy spots, however, is that they tend to have reduced blood flow, and insulin does not absorb properly—if at all. Avoid giving insulin into these areas. Spreading your injection and infusion sites over a large area of skin should help prevent the development of lipodystrophy. And with the exception of NPH and regular, insulin may be given in a variety of body parts without altering the absorption rate.

Missed Injections

Missed or omitted injections are another potential cause of an insulin deficiency. Missing an occasional meal bolus will not typically cause the body to become totally devoid of insulin, but missed basal insulin injections or repeated missed boluses can have serious consequences.

Prevention: Plan to take your basal insulin at about the same time each day. If possible, combine it with another activity, such as brushing your teeth, taking oral medication, or eating a certain meal. Getting into a routine is the best way to ensure that you will not miss critical basal insulin injections. Some blood glucose meters can be programmed with scheduled reminders to check blood sugar or take a bolus. Users of the latest insulin pumps can avoid missing boluses by programming "missed bolus reminders" at key times of day. Those who take injections might have an easier time remembering to bolus if they take blood sugars at each meal/snack time and keep written records. Those who consistently bolus *before* eating are less like to forget compared to those who bolus during or after meals.

Gaps in Coverage

An insulin program that has gaps in insulin coverage or is grossly deficient in the total amount of insulin could also induce ketone production and ketoacidosis.

Prevention: Questioning your doctor's insulin dosage recommendations is reasonable if (1) there is no basal insulin component to your program, or (2) the total amount of insulin for the day is less than 0.5

units per kilogram of your body weight if you have type 1 diabetes or less than 0.25 units per kilogram of your body weight if you have type 2 diabetes.

Insulin Pump Malfunction

Insulin pump therapy opens the door to ketoacidosis in the event of a problem with insulin delivery, absorption, or action. With no intermediate- or long-acting insulin in the body, pumpers rely on the pump's delivery of basal insulin in the form of tiny pulses of rapid-acting insulin. Any interruption in insulin delivery can result in a sharp rise in blood sugar and ketone production starting as soon as three hours after the last bit of insulin was infused. This can be caused by any of the following:

- tubing or infusion set clogs
- leaks where the cartridge connects to the tubing
- air pockets in the tubing
- spoilage of the insulin in the pump
- dislodgement of the canula/infusion set tube from the skin
- not connecting the tube completely at the infusion site
- improper or insufficient priming
- extended pump suspension
- extended disconnection or forgetting to reconnect
- lack of insulin absorption or leakage at the infusion site

Prevention: The first and most important step in preventing ketoacidosis when using an insulin pump is early detection of a problem. This starts with frequent blood sugar checks, followed by ketone checks with any unusually high blood sugar levels. The absence of ketones indicates that the high reading is probably due to insufficient insulin coverage for food eaten recently. The presence of ketones indicates either an illness/infection or, more likely, a problem with the pump's insulin delivery. The troubleshooting process is shown in Figure 9-6:

Figure 9-6. Prevention of DKA when using an insulin pump

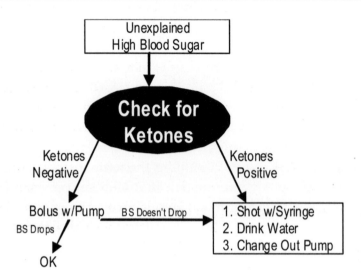

Three steps should reverse the problem if ketones are present.

1. Give an injection of insulin using a syringe, using your normal correction formula to determine the dose. Giving the injection into muscle will help bring your blood sugar down faster and ensure that it absorbs completely.
2. Drink as much water as possible.
3. Change your pump's cartridge, tubing, and infusion set, using a fresh vial of insulin.

Failure to correct the problem could result in ketoacidosis in just a few hours. To prevent insulin delivery problems with your pump, be sure to do the following:

- Limit your disconnection and suspension periods to no more than an hour at a time. If you must disconnect for more than an hour, reconnect hourly and bolus an amount equal to the basal insulin that you missed in the previous hour.

- Check your infusion site and tubing at least once daily. If the infusion set tape is peeling loose or if you spot any blood in the canula or any redness/irritation on your skin, replace the infusion set immediately.
- Check for air pockets in the tubing. If you spot any, disconnect and prime until the air has been purged completely out.
- If you smell insulin or detect moisture around any of the joints where the tubing connects to the pump or infusion set, replace them immediately.
- If your pump alerts you of a tubing/infusion set clog ("no delivery," "occlusion," "blockage detected"), replace your cartridge, tubing, and infusion set immediately. Do not just jiggle your infusion set and attempt to bolus again. Pumps only detect clogs after a significant amount of pressure has built up. Jiggling may temporarily help insulin flow through, but the problem is likely to reoccur.
- Change your cartridge as soon as possible after you receive your "low cartridge" warning. This minimizes the risk that your cartridge will run out completely.
- Do not wear an infusion set in the same place for more than three days. Site problems occur much more often after three days of set usage.
- Rotate sites in an organized fashion. Simply going from right side to left side repeatedly may result in the overuse of two sites. Instead, stay on one side of your body for several site changes, moving just a couple of inches (4–6 cm) each time. Here is an example.

Left side	Right side
1 2 3	12 11 10
6 5 4	13 14 15
7 8 9	18 17 16

Symptoms and Treatment of DKA

Everyone with diabetes who uses insulin should have a way to test for ketones. You can perform ketone testing by way of a urine dipstick or a fingerstick blood sample. (See Chapter 10 for ketone testing supply options.) Positive ketones are indicated by either urine testing that indicates small or more ketones (>15 mg/dl) or blood testing that indicates the presence of ß-Hydroxybutyrate (>0.5 mmol/l).

Be sure to have fresh ketone testing supplies on hand at all times—including when you travel. Ketostix in vials are only good for six months after you have opened the vial. Individually foil-wrapped ketostix are good until their expiration date. Ketone test strips for blood testing are also foil wrapped, but once again, they are only good until the expiration date stamped on the package.

The presence of ketones in the blood is referred to as "ketosis"; the presence of ketones in the urine is "ketonuria." Ketosis and ketonuria are usually—but not always—accompanied by elevated blood sugar, thirst, and excessive urination. This is a precursor to the more severe state of DKA. Symptoms of DKA are more pronounced. With DKA, you are likely to be nauseated or vomiting. Your breathing may be very deep, and you could have a fruity odor on your breath as your lungs try to eliminate ketones when you exhale. You will likely be dehydrated due to all the urination, which is a result of the very high blood sugars. This will give you dry skin, intense thirst, and a dry mouth. Your vision may also be blurry; headache and muscle aches are common.

Call your doctor immediately if you have ketones in your blood or urine, or if you are experiencing these types of symptoms. Although fluids and insulin are the preferred form of treatment, DKA is not something that you can treat on your own. The severe dehydration that accompanies DKA usually keeps insulin from absorbing properly from below the skin. Nausea and vomiting may also limit the amount of water you can consume. Treatment of DKA almost always requires a visit to an emergency room for intravenous administration of insulin, water, and electrolytes. The acidity of your blood will have to be monitored very carefully at the hospital to prevent coma or death. The length of your hospital stay will vary depending on the severity of the DKA, but expect to be there for at least a day or two.

There are a few things that you can do on your own prior to hospitalization. Try to eat light, easy-to-digest carbohydrates and drink at least eight ounces of liquid per hour. Diluted orange juice is a good choice because it replaces fluids as well as potassium that is lost with excess urination. Check your blood sugar and ketones every couple hours, and report the information to your doctor.

Remember: They don't call it "insulin-dependent" diabetes for nothing. We depend on insulin to stay alive. DKA causes more than 80 percent of hospital admissions for people with insulin-dependent diabetes. Practice the preventive measures described above, and stay in close contact with your health care team at the first signs of trouble. Diabetes management is truly a team effort!

Chapter Highlights

Hypoglycemia is a major limiting factor in intensive diabetes control.

- Mild and moderate lows should be self-treatable. Severe hypoglycemia requires glucagon or intravenous dextrose.
- Loss of hypoglycemia symptoms (hypoglycemia unawareness) can be reversed by preventing lows for several weeks.
- Implement strategies to prevent hypoglycemia if you are experiencing more than a few lows per week.
- Taking bolus insulin earlier and/or applying strategies to slow the digestion of your meals can help you minimize after-meal blood sugar spikes.
- A complete lack of insulin in the body can lead to diabetic ketoacidosis (DKA).
- Checking for ketones at the first sign of an unexplained high and administering insulin and fluids if ketones are present can help prevent DKA.

10

Resources for Everything and Anything Diabetes

Giving Support, Getting Support

Feeling the ups and downs of blood sugar swings, handling the incessant responsibilities of managing a chronic disease, trying to make sense out of a highly imperfect science, and facing the grim reality that, despite all your best efforts, serious health problems may be in your future—living with diabetes can be a frustrating and sometimes frightening experience. At times it can also make you feel very much alone.

If you have ever felt the need to reach out to someone who understands how you feel—someone who has *been there*—support networks may be just the answer. Even if you don't feel the need to receive support yourself, the act of giving support to others is worth its weight in gold. Nothing will make you feel better and enrich your life more than helping others.

Opportunities for giving and getting support are widespread—both in-person and on the Internet. And the beauty of it is that you can find groups that are general and diverse or highly specialized.

For an in-person type of support group, your local hospital or diabetes treatment center is a good place to start. If there is a diabetes association office near you, they probably have a listing of support groups in your area. If nothing exists near you or if what exists fails to meet your needs, consider starting a group of your own. Post fliers at doctors' offices and let your local diabetes association chapters know so that they can share the information with their members. Have the meeting at your home or at a centrally located restaurant. You could also ask a social worker at a nearby hospital if there is a room you can use. Each meeting should include plenty of networking/socializing time, but also try to have at least one pertinent topic to address. Have a sign-in sheet so that you can compile a mail and e-mail list for future meetings.

Do not go overboard in terms of expenses for the meetings. Remember: The people in attendance are the highlight. Light snacks and beverages are more than enough. As the group grows you might consider bringing in guest speakers from various hospitals or pharmaceutical companies and ask them to sponsor the meeting by covering your out-of-pocket costs.

If face-to-face groups are not feasible because of space, distance, or your desire for confidentiality, consider participating in or starting a chat room or group on the Internet. Although information derived from online groups may not always be 100 percent accurate, you can still gain an emotional lift from conversing with other people facing similar challenges.

Resources are not limited to mutual support–type programs. There is also an assortment of clinical support, associations, media/publications, government entities, books, product manufacturers, and mail-order suppliers ready to serve you. Below is a list of some of the resources we've found to be highly useful.

Integrated Diabetes Services

Here's my chance to "toot my own horn." My practice, Integrated Diabetes Services, is a worldwide leader in one-on-one consulting for people who use insulin. Diabetes coaching services for both children and adults are available in-person and remotely via phone and the Internet. Our team of highly committed Certified Diabetes Educators (most of whom have diabetes themselves) focuses on improving blood sugar control, teaching advanced self-management skills, and working with you to reach your individual goals. If you're ready to take your diabetes management to the next level, we provide the care, attention, and expertise you've been looking for. Call 877-735-3648, or visit www.integrateddiabetes.com.

Type 1 University

T1U (www.type1university.com) features advanced online courses for insulin users and parents/caregivers of insulin users. Each forty- to sixty-minute class is available live (via webex) or in prerecorded format, accessible on any computer or mobile device with Internet access, so you can participate from the comfort and convenience of your home or office. Enroll in an individual class or a group of courses. Class topics include:

- mastering pump therapy
- advanced carb counting
- blood glucose control during sports and exercise
- weight loss for insulin users
- getting the most from your continuous glucose monitor
- after-meal glucose control
- hypoglycemia prevention and treatment
- fine-tuning basal insulin
- managing pregnancy with type 1 diabetes
- optimizing Symlin therapy

Other Sources of Diabetes Management Consulting

The International Diabetes Center (Minneapolis, MN)
www.idcdiabetes.org; 888-825-6315; international:
1-952-993-3393
Joslin Diabetes Center (Boston, MA)
www.joslin.org; 800-567-5461; 617-309-2400

Barbara Davis Center for Childhood Diabetes (Aurora, CO)
www.barbaradaviscenter.org; 303-724-2323

Dietitian Locator: Contact the American Dietetic Association at 800-877-1600, or visit www.eatright.org/public (click on the "find a nutrition professional" icon).

Diabetes Educator Locator: Visit the American Association of Diabetes Educators at http://www.diabeteseducator.org /DiabetesEducation/Find.html.

Associations/Organizations

American Association of Diabetes Educators (AADE)
800-338-3633
www.aadenet.org

American Association of Kidney Patients
800-749-2257
www.aakp.org

American Chronic Pain Association
800-533-3231
www.theacpa.org

American Diabetes Association (ADA)
800-232-3472
www.diabetes.org

American Dietetic Association (also ADA)
800-877-1600
www.eatright.org

American Foundation for the Blind
800-232-5463
www.afb.org

American Heart Association
800-242-8721
www.amhrt.org

Amputee Coalition of America
888-267-5669
www.amputee-coalition.org

Celiac Society
www.celiacsociety.com
Celiac Sprue Association/USA
402-558-0600
www.csaceliacs.org
Diabetes Camping Association (DCA)
256-883-2556
www.diabetescamps.org
Diabetes Exercise and Sports Association (DESA)
800-898-4322
www.diabetes-exercise.org
Friends with Diabetes (Jewish)
845-352-7532
www.friendswithdiabetes.org
Gluten Intolerance Group of North America
206-246-6652
www.gluten.net
International Association for Medical Assistance to Travelers (IAMAT)
716-754-4883
www.iamat.org
Jewish Diabetes Association (JDA)
718-787-4532
www.jewishdiabetes.org
Juvenile Diabetes Research Foundation (JDRF) ·
800-533-2873
www.jdrf.org
National Center on Physical Activity and Disability
www.ncpad.org
National Diabetes Education Program
800-GET-LEVEL
www.niddk.nih.gov/health/diabetes/ndep/ndep.htm
National Diabetes Information Clearinghouse
800-860-8747
www.niddk.nih.gov/health/diabetes/ndc.htmm

National Federation of the Blind Materials Resource Center
  410-659-9314
  www.nfb.org
National Kidney Foundation
  800-622-9010
  www.kidney.org
National Institute of Dental and Craniofacial Research
  301-402-7364
  www.nidcr.nih.gov
National Institute of Diabetes and Digestive and Kidney Diseases
  301-496-3583
  www.niddk.nih.gov
National Institutes of Health
  301-496-4261
  www.nih.gov
National Library Service for the Blind and Physically Handicapped
  800-424-8567
  www.lcweb.loc.gov/nls
Neuropathy Association
  800-247-6968
  www.neuropathy.org
Taking Control of Your Diabetes (TCOYD)
  www.tcoyd.org;
TrialNet
  www.diabetestrialnet.org
  e-mail: trialnetinfo@epi.usf.edu

Financial Resources

There are many programs available to help offset the cost of diabetes care.

Medicare is a government-sponsored program for people over age sixty-five as well as younger people with serious health problems such as kidney failure. Medicare covers blood glucose monitors, test strips, lancets, insulin pumps/supplies, therapeutic shoes, glaucoma screenings, flu and pneumonia vaccines, and limited counseling by some registered dietitians and Certified Diabetes Educators. Medicare Part D provides prescription drug benefits for items such as insulin and oral diabetes medications. For eligibility information, call the Centers for Medicare and Medicaid Services at 1-800-633-4227, or visit www.medicare.gov.

Medicare also offers a database of public and private *prescription drug assistance programs* at www.medicare.gov/Prescription/Home.asp. The Cost Containment Research Institute (202-318-0770; www.institute-dc.org) provides a similar list. Another website, www.needymeds.com, provides up-to-date information on nearly two hundred patient assistance programs run by drug manufacturers.

Medicaid is a health assistance program sponsored by each individual state. Eligibility is based on your income level. Medicaid recipients may qualify for full or partial coverage for select types of diabetes medications and blood glucose monitors/strips. For information, contact the Department of Human Services in the government pages of your phone book.

CHIP is the Children's Health Insurance Program provided by each state. It is for children whose families earn too much to qualify for Medicaid but too little to afford private health insurance. For information, call 877-543-7669, or visit www.insurekidsnow.gov.

PCIP is the preexisting condition insurance plan, established by the Affordable Care Act and administered by the U.S. Department of Health and Human Services. It provides a health coverage option for children and adults who have been locked out of the insurance market because of a preexisting health condition. For information or to apply, find your state at www.pcip.gov, or call 866-717-5826.

The Bureau of Primary Health Care (also called the Hill-Burton Program) offers professional medical care regardless of insurance status or ability to pay. For a directory of local primary health care centers, call 800-400-2742, or visit www.bphc.hrsa.gov.

The VA (Department of Veteran Affairs) runs hospitals and clinics for veterans who need treatment for service-related ailments and/or financial aid. To find out more about VA health benefits, call 800-827-1000, or visit www.va.gov.

WIC (Women, Infants and Children) is founded on the premise that healthy eating is an essential component of diabetes self-care. With this in mind, women with preexisting diabetes who become pregnant as well as those who develop gestational diabetes may be eligible for assistance with grocery costs if certain criteria are met. For more information call WIC Headquarters at 703-305-2746, or visit www.fns.usda.gov/wic.

Together Rx is a program in which people who have no prescription coverage and are not eligible for Medicare may be able to obtain a free Together Rx Access Card. Using the card can save you 25 to 40 percent on a select list of brand-name and generic drugs/supplies (including insulin, oral diabetes medications, meters, and test strips). For qualification information and a list of covered drugs, call 800-444-4106, or visit www.togetherrxaccess.com.

Lilly Cares is a patient assistance program for users of Eli Lilly insulin and other medications. Free insulin is provided by way of coupons supplied to your physician. Lilly Cares is open to legal U.S. residents who cannot qualify for government-sponsored programs, do not have private insurance, and fall below a certain income level. For more information, call 800-545-6962, or visit www.lillycares.com.

Novo Nordisk offers a Patient Assistance Program that provides free insulin, pen needles, and glucagon kits for those who cannot qualify for government-sponsored programs, do not have private insurance, and fall below a certain income level. For more information, call 866-310-7549.

Aventis Pharmaceuticals also offers a Patient Assistance Program that provides free insulin to those who cannot qualify for government-sponsored programs, do not have private insurance, and fall below a certain income level. For more information, call 800-221-4025.

Medtronic, makers of insulin pumps and pump supplies, offers financial assistance for those who use or are looking to use insulin pumps. Contact the Charles Ray III Diabetes Foundation at 919-303-6949, or e-mail chuck@charlesray.g12.com.

Glucose Test Strip manufacturers often provide copay cards for users of their blood glucose meters. The copay cards either reduce or eliminate copays associated with test strip purchases. There are usually no income or insurance eligibility limits. For details, call the toll-free number on the back of your glucose meter.

In the United States, each state has its own *Attorney General's Office* whose job is to enforce laws and regulations of that particular state. Since most healthcare standards are enacted and governed by each state, the Attorney General's Office can come to your aid if you feel that you are being dealt with unfairly by your health insurance, healthcare providers, pharmaceutical company, or a medical device manufacturer. Check in the white pages of your phone book, or search online for the attorney general office for your particular state for contact information.

Media and Publications

Countdown (published by the Juvenile Diabetes Research Foundation)
800-533-2873
www.jdrf.org

Diabetes Forecast (published by the American Diabetes Association)
800-806-7801
www.diabetes.org/diabetesforecast/

Diabetes Health
415-883-1990
www.diabeteshealth.com

Diabetes Living Today (radio)
http://www.diabeteslivingtoday.com

Diabetes Monitor
www.diabetesmonitor.com

Diabetes Self-Management (published by Rapaport Publishing)
800-234-0923
www.diabetesselfmanagement.com

Diabetic Cooking (published by Publications International)
800-777-5582
www.fbnr.com

dLife (TV, web portal, and mobile)
  203-454-6985
  www.dLife.com; email: info@dlife.com
TCOYD (TV) with Steven Edelman, MD
  http://tcoyd.org/series-television/tcoyd-tv.html

Fab Websites

www.1happydiabetic.com/
  Just the right formula for a positive attitude
www.bd.com/us/diabetes/page.aspx?cat=7001
  BD (Becton-Dickinson)'s Diabetes Learning Center
www.childrenwithdiabetes.com
  Unlimited resources for kids and parents
www.closeconcerns.com
  A consultancy devoted to the business of diabetes
www.deo.ucsf.edu
  University of California Online Diabetes Teaching Center
www.diabetesdaily.com
  Diabetes news, tools, community, and blogs
www.diabetesincontrol.com
  Free weekly news and information for diabetes
  health professionals
www.diabetesnet.com
  Diabetes information, research findings, and discounted
  diabetes products
www.diabetessisters.org
  Focused on women and women's issues
www.diabeticmommy.com
  For expectant and recent moms
www.diabetesmine.com
  A "gold mine" of straight talk and encouragement for people
  living with diabetes

www.diabeticinvestor.com
  David Kliff's business/investor report on the diabetes industry
  (pay site)
www.diatribe.us/home.php
  Research and product news for the well-informed
  person with diabetes
www.friendswithdiabetes.org
  Incorporating diabetes into a Jewish lifestyle
www.hypoactive.org
  Promoting an active lifestyle for PWDs in Australia
www.insulin-pumpers.org
  For pump users and those interested in pump therapy
www.insulindependence.org
  Inspiring fitness goals, adaptive strategies for sport, and
  recreational programs
www.integrateddiabetes.com
  Gary Scheiner's company; features several free
  self-management tools
www.juvenation.org
  A network hub of type 1 diabetes communities, created by JDRF
www.mendosa.com/diabetes.htm
  David Mendosa's website (various resources and information)
www.parentingdiabetickids.com
  For parents of kids with diabetes
www.phrendo.com
  Make personal connections with diabetic athletes
www.sixuntilme.com
  Kerry Sparling: Diabetes doesn't define me,
  but it helps explain me
www.studentswithdiabetes.com
  Organized by Nicole Johnson (Miss America 1999)
  and provides a community for college students with diabetes
www.thebetesnow.com
  Creative use of media in exploring the world of diabetes

www.thecgmresourcecenter.com
 The place to go for continuous glucose monitoring insight, education, and tools
www.thediabetesoc.com
 Featured bloggers of the week
www.thediabetesresource.com
 Your ultimate guide to everything diabetes related
www.triabetes.org
 Athletes take on triathlons while mentoring "triabuddies"
www.tudiabetes.org
 A community of people touched by diabetes, run by the Diabetes Hands Foundation
www.type1university.com
 The online school of higher learning for insulin users

Blogs

http://25unitstogo.wordpress.com/
 Harry's sarcastic outlook on life with diabetes
http://www.act1diabetes.org/
 Blogs from various adults coping with type 1 diabetes
http://badpancreas.wordpress.com/
 "Typical type 1" Jacquie expresses herself in the most creative ways
http://christophermassa.blogspot.com/
 A blog about photography and pushing oneself through sport
http://www.d-mom.com/
 The ups and downs of life with a diabetic child
http://diabetesaliciousness.blogspot.com/
 Kelly Kunik tackles diabetes through humor, diabetes ownership, and advocacy
http://www.diabetesdaily.com/farrell/
 Bernard Farrell's diabetes technology blog

http://www.diabetesstories.com/stories_blog/
Author Riva Greenberg's inspiring and informative posts

http://diabetestalkfest.com
Gina Capone: your diabetes BFF

http://dorkabetic.blogspot.com
Hannah's dorky life with diabetes

http://www.healthcentral.com/diabeteens/
Teen blog hosted by HealthCentral

http://lemonlemonade.wordpress.com/
The journey of Allison Blass and her life
with type 1 diabetes

http://living-in-progress.com
Ginger Vieira's upbeat for 'betes sake blog

http://www.ninjabetic.com/
. . . because it takes being a ninja to live successfully
with diabetes

http://scottsdiabetes.com/
Scott Johnson's struggles, successes, and
everything in between

http://blog.sstrumello.com/
Scott Strumello's no-holds-barred look at the
science of diabetes

http://sugabetic.wordpress.com/
In the South, you don't have diabetes; you have
"the Suga," says Sarah.

http://www.thebuttercompartment.com/
Hosted by Lee Ann Thill, diabetes blogger and art therapist

http://www.thegirlsguidetodiabetes.com/
Sysy Morales's offbeat observations for girls living with diabetes

http://thelifeofadiabetic.com/
Chris Stocker's attempt to live a normal life with diabetes

http://tobesugarfree.com/
Christopher Snider says, "What good is an
incurable disease if you can't share it?"

Recommended Reading

*Available at the Integrated Diabetes Services online store: www.integrated diabetes.com/webstore/

The 10 Keys to Helping Your Child Grow Up with Diabetes*
By Tim Wysocki, PhD, one of the top mental health experts in diabetes. An excellent resource for helping parents face problems and deal with the feelings and situations that impact their everyday lives.

50 Secrets of the Longest Living People with Diabetes*
By Sheri E. Colberg, PhD and Steven V. Edelman, MD, this book shares interviews with more than fifty people who have thrived with diabetes for as many as eighty-four years. It offers practical advice to escape or control serious diabetic complications and live a more vibrant life with diabetes.

Balancing Pregnancy with Pre-Existing Diabetes*
By Cheryl Alkon. A down-to-earth guide for diabetic mothers-to-be. Author Cheryl Alkon has lived with type 1 diabetes for thirty-one years and brings a wealth of understanding to the subject. It includes firsthand accounts by diabetic women sharing their pregnancy-related experiences. Topics include what is diabetes; finding the right doctor; strategies to successfully conceive; the first, second, and third trimesters; labor and delivery; and balancing the woman's health needs with those of her child.

Caring for the Diabetic Soul*
ADA publication. This is an inspirational guide for people with diabetes to achieve and maintain a healthy emotional balance.

Complete Book of Food Counts, 8th Ed.
By Corinne T. Netzer. Featuring thousands of new listings—and thousands more choices than ever before—this completely revised book features an up-to-date reference on generic and brand-name foods *plus* the latest gourmet, health, and ethnic foods.

Complete Guide to Carb Counting
An ADA publication, written by Hope Warshaw and Karmeen Kulkarni. This is the A–Z guide to carbohydrate counting for diabetes, whether you want to learn basic or advanced carb counting.

Diabetes Burnout: What to Do
When You Can't Take It Anymore

By famed psychologist Dr. William Polonsky. Living with diabetes is hard. It's easy to get discouraged, frustrated, and burned out. Here's an author that understands the emotional rollercoaster and gives you the tools you need to keep from being overwhelmed, addressing such issues as dealing with friends and family as well as how you can better handle the stress for better health.

Diabetic Athlete's Handbook:
Your Guide to Peak Performance

By renowned diabetes/exercise specialist Dr. Sheri Colberg. Contains examples from over 350 diabetic exercisers, an additional fifteen sports and activities, examples from type 1, 1.5, and 2 diabetic athletes using the newest medications and regimens, chapters on thinking like an athlete and sports injury treatment and prevention, ten athlete profiles, along with the latest research on diabetes and exercise, fitness, nutrition, and more.

The Doctor's Pocket Calorie, Fat & Carbohydrate Counter*

By Family Health Publications. This is a compact paperback with a very comprehensive listing of carb content of common foods, ethnic foods, restaurant foods, and beverages. It is indexed for easy searching and is also available in electronic form through www.CalorieKing.com.

Eating Mindfully: How to End Mindless Eating and
Enjoy a Balanced Relationship with Food*

By Susan Albers, PsyD. Learn how to end mindless eating and enjoy a balanced relationship with food.

Get Control of Your Blood Sugar*

By Gary Scheiner, MS, CDE. A complete guide to help those with type 2 diabetes to eliminate highs and lows, decrease the risk of complications, and lower the odds of developing diabetes if you are prediabetic.

Guide to Healthy Restaurant Eating

By Hope Warshaw. This guide helps you avoid the pitfalls of restaurant eating and develop skills and strategies to eat and enjoy healthy restaurant meals.

Insulin Pump Therapy Demystified:
An Essential Guide for Everyone Pumping Insulin*
By Gabrielle Kaplan-Meyer. Many who stand to benefit from the pump are put off by not fully understanding the device, and many already using it don't have anyone with whom to compare notes about its use. *Demystified* offers insight into the day-to-day challenges—and rewards—of life with an insulin pump. Drawing on interviews with more than seventy-five pump users, including Nicole Johnson, Miss America 1999, as well as diabetes experts, *Demystified* discusses how the pump affects your sex life, dealing with money issues, finding support, counting carbohydrates, and much more.

The New Glucose Revolution:
The Authoritative Guide to the Glycemic Index
By Dr. Jennie Brand-Miller, Thomas M. S. Wolever, Kaye Foster-Powell, and Stephen Colagiuri. This book focuses on the role of glycemic index in blood sugar control, satiety, weight control, and proper nutrition. It also includes extensive glycemic index and glycemic load listings.

Pumping Insulin: Everything You Need for
Success on a Smart Insulin Pump*
By John Walsh and Ruth Roberts, two of the world's foremost authorities on insulin pump therapy. This book covers pump basics, troubleshooting, daily living, and managing blood sugars with an insulin pump. It also includes log sheets, recording charts, and carb factor listings.

Real-Life Guide to Diabetes:
Practical Answers to Your Diabetes Problems
By Hope S. Warshaw, RD and Joy Pape, RN. This one-of-a-kind book uses an easy-to-search format to help you find the answers to your most pressing questions quickly and easily.

The Ultimate Guide to Accurate Carb Counting:
Featuring the Tools and Techniques Used by the Experts*
By Gary Scheiner, MS, CDE. This all-in-one resource for effectively keeping track of your carb intake teaches both basic and advanced carb counting techniques. It includes an expansive carb-counting resource list with fiber listings, ethnic foods, party/festival foods, and nearly one hundred national and regional restaurant chains.

Your Diabetes Science Experiment
By Ginger Vieira, a type 1 diabetic and record-setting competitive power-lifter. This is a book for people with type 1, 1.5, and 2 diabetes who want to gain a deeper understanding of how the basic science of the human body impacts blood sugar levels and insulin needs.

Products

Insulin and Injectables

Amylin Pharmaceuticals
    (pramlintide/Symlin, exenatide/Byetta)
    800-349-8919
    www.symlin.com
    800-868-1190
    www.byetta.com
Eli Lilly and Company (lispro/Humalog,
    Humulin regular and NPH insulin, glucagon)
    800-545-5979
    www.lillydiabetes.com
Novo Nordisk Pharmaceuticals
    (aspart/Novolog and Novorapid, detemir/Levemir, Novolin
    regular and NPH insulin, liraglutide/Victoza, glucagen)
    800-727-6500
    www.novonordisk-us.com
Sanofi-Aventis (glargine/Lantus and glulisine/Apidra insulin)
    800-981-2491
    www.lantus.com/; www.apidra.com

Syringes and Pen Needles

Abbott (Precision Sure-Dose)
    800-252-6782
    www.abbottdiabetescare.com

Allison Medical (SureComfort)
800-886-1618
www.allisonmedical.com

Becton Dickinson / BD (UltraFine, UltraFine II, UltraFine III, UltraFine Short, Nano)
888-232-2737
www.bddiabetes.com

Can-Am Care (Monject Ultra Comfort, ReliOn, ClickFine)
800-461-7448
www.canamcare.com

Novo Nordisk (NovoFine)
800-727-6500
www.novolog.com/devices-alt_devices.asp

Owen Mumford (Unifine)
(UK) 01993 812021
www.owenmumford.com/us/range/30/unifine-pentips

Ypsomed AG (ClickFine)
(Switzerland) +41 (0) 34 424 41 11
www.ypsomed.com

Insulin Pens

Eli Lilly (Kwikpen, Luxura HD, Memoir)
800-545-5979
www.lillydiabetes.com

Novo Nordisk (Flexpen, Novopen3, NovoPen Junior)
800-727-6500
www.novonordisk-us.com

Owen Mumford (Autopen Classic)
(UK) 01993 812021
www.owenmumford.com/en/range/6/autopen

Sanofi-Aventis (Solostar)
800-981-2491
www.lantus.com/; www.apidra.com

Pump Manufacturers

Animas Corp. (2020 and Ping insulin pumps)
877-937-7867
www.animascorp.com

Asante Solutions (Pearl Insulin Pump)
408-716-5600
www.asantesolutions.com

Insulet Corp. (OmniPod)
781-457-5000 (outside US: 781-457-5098)
http://www.myomnipod.co

Medtronic Diabetes
(Paradigm Revel insulin pumps)
800-646-4633
www.minimed.com

Roche/Disetronic
(Accu-Chek Spirit and Solo Micropump)
800-280-7801
www.accu-chekinsulinpumps.com

Sooil Development USA (DANA Diabecare IIS)
866-747-6645
www.sooilusa.com

Infusion Set Manufacturers

ICU Medical (Orbit)
800-824-7890
www.icumed.com/orbit-90.asp

Medtronic Diabetes (Sof-Set, Sure-T)
800-646-4633
www.minimed.com/products/infusionsets/index.html

Roche (FlexLink, Rapid-D)
800-280-7801
www.accu-chekinsulinpumps.com

Unomedical (Comfort/Tender/Silhouette, Quick-Set, Inset, Mio, Contact)
(Denmark) 011 45 4816 7000
www.infusion-set.com

Pump Accessories

Angel Bear Pump Stuff
877-586-PUMP
www.angelbearpumpstuff.com

Funky Pumpers
(UK) 0845 009 4014
www.funkypumpers.com

Groovy Patches
877-813-9369
www.groovypatches.com

Pump Wear Inc.
866-470-PUMP
www.pumpwearinc.com

Unique Pump Accessories
800-831-8929
www.uniaccs.com

Injection Ports

Patton Medical (I-Port)
877-763-7678
www.i-port.com

Unomedical (Insuflon)
(Denmark) 011 45 4816 7000
www.infusion-set.com

Glucose Meters

Abbott Diabetes Care (Freestyle and Precision meters)
888-522-5226
www.abbottdiabetescare.com

AgaMatrix (Wavesense meters)
866-906-4197
www.wavesense.info

Bayer (Breeze, Contour, and Didget meters)
800-348-8100
www.simplewins.com

Diagnostic Devices (Prodigy meters)
800-243-2636
www.prodigymeter.com

LifeScan (One Touch meters)
800-227-8862
www.onetouchdiabetes.com

Nova Biomedical (Nova Max meters)
800-681-7390
www.novacares.com

Roche (Accu-Chek meters)
800-858-8072
www.accu-chek.com/us

Lancing Devices, Lancets

Bayer (Microlet Vaculance)
800-348-8100
www.simplewins.com

Becton Dickinson/BD (UltraFine lancets)
888-232-2737
www.bddiabetes.com

Health Innovation Ideas (Tiniboy lancets)
888-417-5264
www.tiniboy.com

Lifescan (One Touch Delica)
800-227-8862
www.onetouchdiabetes.com

Palco Labs (Auto Lancet, Auto Lancet Mini)
831-430-1603
www.palcolabs.com

Roche (Accu-Chek Softclix and Multiclix)
  800-858-8072
  www.accu-chek.com/us

Continuous Glucose Monitors

Abbott (Freestyle Navigator)
  510-749-5400
  www.freestylenavigator.com
Dexcom (Dexcom Seven Plus)
  877-339-2664
  www.dexcom.com
Medtronic (Paradigm Revel Real-Time Pump,
  Guardian System, and iPro)
  (800) 646-4633
  www.minimed.com

Downloading Software

Abbott: CoPilot
  www.abbottdiabetescare.com
AgaMatrix: Zero Click
  www.wavesense.info/zero-click
Animas: Diasend
  www.diasend.com/animas
Bayer: Glucofacts Deluxe
  www.simplewins.com
Dexcom: DM3
  877-339-2664
  www.dexcom.com
Home Diagnostics: True Manager
  http://homediagnosticsinc.com
Lifescan: One Touch Zoom DMS
  www.lifescan.com/products/otdms/
Medtronic: Carelink
  www.carelink.minimed.com

Nova Max (BD Interactiv)
www.bd.com/diabetes/
ReliOn: My Care Team
800-631-0076
www.mycareteam.com
Roche: Accu-Chek 360°
www.accu-chek.com/us

Home A1c

Bayer (A1c Now)
800-348-8100
http://www.simplewins.com/sections/Monitor/meters/a1c/overview
Heritage Labs (Appraise A1c test kit)
888-764-2384
www.appraisetests.com/p-1-blood-collection-kit-a1c
Walmart (ReliOn A1c test kit)
www.walmart.com/ip/ReliOn-A1c-Test/10575934

Ketone Testing

Abbott Diabetes Care (Precision Xtra blood ketone meter)
888-522-5226
www.abbottdiabetescare.com
Bayer Health Care (ketostix and ketodiastix)
800-348-8100
www.bayercarediabetes.com
Nova Biomedical (Nova Max Plus blood ketone meter)
800-681-7390
www.novacares.com

Hypoglycemia Treatment

Can-Am Care (Dex4 products)
888-400-9770
www.dex4.com

PBM Products (GlucoBurst)
    800-485-9809
    www.glucoburst.com
Paddock Laboratories (glucose tubes)
    800-328-5113
    www.glutose.com
ReliOn
    800-461-7448
    www.relion.com

Supply Cases

Cooler Concepts (Frio cooling wallets)
    866-690-3746
    www.coolerconcept.com
Fifty50 Medical (SportKids supply cases)
    800-746-7505
    www.fifty50pharmacy.com
Medicool, Inc. (insulated storage/travel cases)
    800-433-2469
    www.medicool.com

Medical Identification

Fifty50 Medical (SportKids ID)
    800-746-7505
    www.fifty50pharmacy.com
Lauren's Hope Medical ID Bracelets
    800-360-8680
    www.laurenshope.com
Medic Alert Foundation
    800-432-5378
    www.medicalert.org
Rescue Me IDs
    866-713-3808
    www.rescuemeIDs.com

Adaptive Devices

BD (Magni-Guide)
888-232-2737
www.bddiabetes.com

Diagnostic Devices (Prodigy talking meters)
800-243-2636
www.prodigymeter.com

LS&S Group (catalog of products for those with visual, hearing, or dexterity limitations)
800-468-4789
www.lssproducts.com

Owen Mumford (Autoject 2)
(UK) 01993 812021
www.owenmumford.com/en/range/8/autoject-2

Suppliers

Byram Healthcare (mail-order diabetes supplies)
877-902-9726
www.byramhealthcare.com

Diabetes Mall (discounted diabetes products)
www.diabetesnet.com

Diabetes Specialty Center (mail-order diabetes supplies)
800-775-4372
www.diabetesspecialty.com

Logsheets

Diabetes Logsheet   Name:_____

Date	6-7 AM	7-8 AM	8-9 AM	9-10 AM	10-11 AM	11-12 N	12-1 PM	1-2 PM	2-3 PM	3-4 PM	4-5 PM	5-6 PM	6-7 PM	7-8 PM	8-9 PM	9-10 PM	10-11 PM	11-12 M	12-1 AM	1-2 AM	2-3 AM	3-4 AM	4-5 AM	5-6 AM
Blood Sugar																								
Grams Carb																								
Insulin																								
Phys. Activity																								
Notes																								

Date	6-7 AM	7-8 AM	8-9 AM	9-10 AM	10-11 AM	11-12 N	12-1 PM	1-2 PM	2-3 PM	3-4 PM	4-5 PM	5-6 PM	6-7 PM	7-8 PM	8-9 PM	9-10 PM	10-11 PM	11-12 M	12-1 AM	1-2 AM	2-3 AM	3-4 AM	4-5 AM	5-6 AM
Blood Sugar																								
Grams Carb																								
Insulin																								
Phys. Activity																								
Notes																								

Date	6-7 AM	7-8 AM	8-9 AM	9-10 AM	10-11 AM	11-12 N	12-1 PM	1-2 PM	2-3 PM	3-4 PM	4-5 PM	5-6 PM	6-7 PM	7-8 PM	8-9 PM	9-10 PM	10-11 PM	11-12 M	12-1 AM	1-2 AM	2-3 AM	3-4 AM	4-5 AM	5-6 AM
Blood Sugar																								
Grams Carb																								
Insulin																								
Phys. Activity																								
Notes																								

Name: _____ **Blood Sugar Patterns** (Review & adjust weekly)

Date	Wake-Up (pre-bkfst)	Pre-Lunch	Afternoon	Pre-Dinner	Bedtime (pre-snack)

# High:					
# OK:					
# Low:					

Changes*: _____

If 3 or more highs, or 2 or more lows, change 1:C ratio at the previous meal or snack!

Insulin Pump User Logsheet   Name: _____

Day/Date	6-7 AM	7-8 AM	8-9 AM	9-10 AM	10-11 AM	11-12 N	12-1 PM	1-2 PM	2-3 PM	3-4 PM	4-5 PM	5-6 PM	6-7 PM	7-8 PM	8-9 PM	9-10 PM	10-11 PM	11-12 M	12-1 AM	1-2 AM	2-3 AM	3-4 AM	4-5 AM	5-6 AM
Blood Sugar																								
Grams Carb																								
Boluses																								
Basal Rates																								
Phys. Activity																								

Notes (set changes, ketone tests, severe lows, etc.):

Day/Date	6-7 AM	7-8 AM	8-9 AM	9-10 AM	10-11 AM	11-12 N	12-1 PM	1-2 PM	2-3 PM	3-4 PM	4-5 PM	5-6 PM	6-7 PM	7-8 PM	8-9 PM	9-10 PM	10-11 PM	11-12 M	12-1 AM	1-2 AM	2-3 AM	3-4 AM	4-5 AM	5-6 AM
Blood Sugar																								
Grams Carb																								
Boluses																								
Basal Rates																								
Phys. Activity																								

Notes (set changes, ketone tests, severe lows, etc.):

Day/Date	6-7 AM	7-8 AM	8-9 AM	9-10 AM	10-11 AM	11-12 N	12-1 PM	1-2 PM	2-3 PM	3-4 PM	4-5 PM	5-6 PM	6-7 PM	7-8 PM	8-9 PM	9-10 PM	10-11 PM	11-12 M	12-1 AM	1-2 AM	2-3 AM	3-4 AM	4-5 AM	5-6 AM
Blood Sugar																								
Grams Carb																								
Boluses																								
Basal Rates																								
Phys. Activity																								

Notes (set changes, ketone tests, severe lows, etc.):

Gary Scheiner, MS, CDE
INTEGRATED DIABETES SERVICES
333 E. Lancaster Ave., Suite 204, Wynnewood, PA 19096
Phone: **(610) 642-6055**   Fax: **(610) 642-8046**

Name: _____

Weekly Diabetes Record

Date:	Breakfast	Snack	Lunch	Snack	Dinner	Snack	Bedtime	Night	Notes
Blood Sugar									
Insulin Dose									
Grams Carb									
Phys. Activity									

Date:	Breakfast	Snack	Lunch	Snack	Dinner	Snack	Bedtime	Night	Notes
Blood Sugar									
Insulin Dose									
Grams Carb									
Phys. Activity									

Date:	Breakfast	Snack	Lunch	Snack	Dinner	Snack	Bedtime	Night	Notes
Blood Sugar									
Insulin Dose									
Grams Carb									
Phys. Activity									

Date:	Breakfast	Snack	Lunch	Snack	Dinner	Snack	Bedtime	Night	Notes
Blood Sugar									
Insulin Dose									
Grams Carb									
Phys. Activity									

Date:	Breakfast	Snack	Lunch	Snack	Dinner	Snack	Bedtime	Night	Notes
Blood Sugar									
Insulin Dose									
Grams Carb									
Phys. Activity									

Date:	Breakfast	Snack	Lunch	Snack	Dinner	Snack	Bedtime	Night	Notes
Blood Sugar									
Insulin Dose									
Grams Carb									
Phys. Activity									

Date:	Breakfast	Snack	Lunch	Snack	Dinner	Snack	Bedtime	Night	Notes
Blood Sugar									
Insulin Dose									
Grams Carb									
Phys. Activity									

Name:	

Weekly Diabetes Record

Date:	Breakfast	Lunch	Dinner	Bedtime	Notes
Blood Sugar					
Food					
Phys. Activity					

Date:	Breakfast	Lunch	Dinner	Bedtime	Notes
Blood Sugar					
Food					
Phys. Activity					

Date:	Breakfast	Lunch	Dinner	Bedtime	Notes
Blood Sugar					
Food					
Phys. Activity					

Date:	Breakfast	Lunch	Dinner	Bedtime	Notes
Blood Sugar					
Food					
Phys. Activity					

Date:	Breakfast	Lunch	Dinner	Bedtime	Notes
Blood Sugar					
Food					
Phys. Activity					

Date:	Breakfast	Lunch	Dinner	Bedtime	Notes
Blood Sugar					
Food					
Phys. Activity					

Date:	Breakfast	Lunch	Dinner	Bedtime	Notes
Blood Sugar					
Food					
Phys. Activity					

©2005 Gary Scheiner MS, CDE – Integrated Diabetes Services (877) 735-3648; (610) 642-6055 www.integrateddiabetes.com

Carb Factors

almonds	.07	bread crumbs	.70
almonds, honey roasted	.14	bread stuffing	.18
apple juice	.11	bread, cornbread	.45
apples, raw	.12	bread, French	.48
applesauce, sweetened	.18	bread, Italian	.47
applesauce, unsweetened	.10	bread, raisin	.48
apricots	.08	bread, white	.47
artichokes	.05	bread, whole-wheat	.39
asparagus, raw	.02	broccoli, raw	.02
bagels, plain	.51	cabbage, raw	.03
baking chocolate	.64	cake, angel food	.56
bananas	.21	cake, chocolate with	
beans, baked, homemade	.15	chocolate frosting	.51
beans, green	.02	cake, chocolate without frosting	.57
beans, kidney	.16	cake, coffeecake	.44
beans, lima	.09	cake, cupcakes	.60
beef jerky	.09	cake, fruitcake	.48
beef stew, canned entrée	.05	cake, pound	.62
beer, light	.10	cake, sponge	.95
beer, regular	.30	candies, butterscotch	.75
biscuits, plain or buttermilk	.47	candies, caramel	.78
blackberries, raw	.07	candies, fudge	.98
blueberries, raw	.11	candies, hard	.93

candies, jellybeans	.68	cheese, cream	.02
candies, M&M	.44	cheese, mozzarella	.02
candies, milk chocolate	.55	cheese, Parmesan, grated	.03
candies, milk chocolate–coated		cheese, ricotta	.05
peanuts	.64	cheese, Swiss	.03
candies, milk chocolate–coated		cherries	.14
raisins	.64	chicken pot pie	.18
candies, semisweet chocolate	.57	chili with beans	.07
carbonated beverage, cola	.10	coleslaw	.10
carbonated beverage, ginger ale	.80	cookies, animal crackers	.73
carrots, baby, raw	.06	cookies, chocolate chip	.64
cashew nuts, dry	.29	cookies, chocolate sandwich	.67
catsup	.25	cookies, graham crackers	.74
cauliflower	.02	cookies, oatmeal	.65
celery	.01	cookies, oatmeal raisin	.64
cereal, All-Bran, Kellogg's	.43	cookies, sugar-free	.65
cereal, Apple Jacks, Kellogg's	.87	corn, sweet, white, raw	.16
cereal, Captain Crunch, Quaker	.82	couscous, cooked	.21
cereal, Cheerios, General Mills	.67	crackers, cheese	.55
cereal, Corn Flakes, Kellogg's	.83	crackers, Matzo	.80
cereal, corn grits	.12	crackers, saltines	.68
cereal, Cream of Wheat	.11	cranberries	.08
cereal, crispy rice	.87	cranberry juice	.14
cereal, Frosted Flakes, Kellogg's	.89	cream puffs (including éclair)	.22
cereal, Frosted Mini-Wheats,		cream, sour	.04
Kellogg's	.71	croissants, butter	.43
cereal, Fruit Loops, Kellogg's	.86	croutons	.68
cereal, Grape-Nuts, Kraft	.72	cucumbers, plain with peel	.01
cereal, Lucky Charms,		daiquiri	.06
General Mills	.79	danish, cinnamon	.43
cereal, oatmeal, Quaker	.14	doughnuts, chocolate glazed	.55
cereal, oats, regular and		doughnuts, plain	.48
quick and instant	.09	eggs, whole, cooked, fried	.01
cereal, Quaker Oats, Quaker	.61	English muffins, whole wheat	.33
cereal, Raisin Bran, Kellogg's	.63	frozen yogurt, chocolate,	
cereal, Rice Krispies, Kellogg's	.85	soft serve	.22
cereal, Shredded Wheat, Kraft	.71	grapefruit, raw	.06
cereal, Wheaties, General Mills	.72	grapes, red or green	.16
cheese, Cheddar	.01	gravy, beef	.04

hummus	.08	plums, raw	.11
ice cream, chocolate	.27	popcorn, air-popped	.62
ice cream, vanilla soft serve	.22	popcorn, caramel-coated	.73
ice cream, vanilla	.23	popcorn, cheese-flavored	.41
kiwifruit	.11	popcorn, oil-popped	.47
lettuce, raw	.01	potato, baked, flesh and skin	.22
macaroni and cheese	.10	potato chips	.48
macaroni, cooked	.27	potato pancakes	.26
mangos, raw	.15	potato salad	.09
melons, cantaloupe	.07	potatoes, French fried	.27
melons, honeydew	.08	potatoes, hash brown	.26
milk, low-fat	.05	potatoes, mashed	.15
muffins, blueberry	.45	potatoes, scalloped	.08
mushrooms, raw	.02	pretzels, hard	.76
noodles, egg	.23	pudding, chocolate	.21
onion rings	.36	raisins, seedless	.75
onions, raw	.06	raspberries, raw	.04
oranges, raw	.09	rice noodles, cooked	.23
oranges, raw with peel	.11	rice, brown	.21
pancakes, plain from recipe	.28	rice, white	.27
peaches, raw	.09	rolls, dinner	.47
peanut butter, smooth	.13	salad dressing, Italian	.10
peanuts, dry-roasted	.13	sherbet, orange	.30
peanuts, Spanish	.08	shrimp, breaded and fried	.11
pears, raw	.12	Rice Krispies Treats	.79
peas, green, raw	.09	soybeans, green	.06
pecans	.04	spaghetti, cooked	.26
peppers, sweet, green, raw	.04	spinach, cooked	.01
pickles, cucumber, dill	.02	squash, summer	.02
pie, apple	.32	squash, winter, butternut	.10
pie, blueberry	.33	strawberries	.04
pie, Boston cream	.41	sweet potato, raw	.21
pie crust, cookie	.62	syrup, maple	.67
pie, pumpkin	.24	taco shells, baked	.54
piña colada	.22	tangerines	.08
pineapple, raw	.11	tomato, paste	.15
pistachio nuts, raw	.17	tomato, raw	.03
pizza, pepperoni	.27	tomato, sauce	.07
pizza, plain	.32	tortilla chips	.57

tortilla chips, nacho-flavored	.57	watermelon	.06
tuna salad	.09	wine, sweet	.11
waffles	.36	wine, table	.01
walnuts	.07	yam, raw	.23

Glycemic Index
of Common Foods

A food's glycemic index value indicates the speed and ease with which it raises blood glucose levels. Higher numbers indicate a fast, sharp rise in blood sugar. Lower numbers indicate a prolonged, gradual rise in blood sugar.

For more information on the GI, check out the following books:

The Low GI Diet Handbook by Dr. Jennie Brand-Miller, Dr. Thomas M. S. Wolever, Kaye Foster-Powell, and Dr. Stephen Colagiuri

The New Glucose Revolution for Diabetes by Dr. Jennie Brand-Miller, Kaye Foster-Powell, Alan W. Barclay, and Dr. Stephen Colagiuri

The Low GI Shopper's Guide to GI Values 2011 by Dr. Jennie Brand-Miller and Kaye Foster-Powell

Bread/Crackers		pumpernickel	51
bagel	72	rye, dark	76
crispbread	81	saltines	74
croissant	67	sourdough	52
French baguette	95	stoned wheat thins	67
graham crackers	74	wheat bread, high fiber	68
hamburger bun	61	white bread	71
kaiser roll	73		
melba toast	70	**Cakes/Cookies/Muffins**	
pita bread	57	angel food cake	67

banana bread	47	Special K	66
blueberry muffin	59	Total	76
chocolate cake	38	waffles	76
corn muffin	102		
cupcake with icing	73	**Combination Foods**	
donut	76	chicken nuggets	46
oat bran muffin	60	fish fingers	38
oatmeal cookies	55	macaroni and cheese	64
pound cake	54	pizza (cheese)	60
shortbread cookies	64	sausages	8
vanilla wafers	77	stuffing	74
		taco shells	68

Candy

chocolate	49	**Dairy**	
jelly beans	80	chocolate milk	34
Lifesavers	70	custard	43
M & M, peanut	33	ice cream, vanilla	62
Nestle Crunch	42	ice cream, chocolate	68
Skittles	69	milk, skim	32
Snickers Bar	40	milk, whole	27
Twix Bar	43	pudding	43
		yogurt, low-fat	33

Cereals/Breakfast

All-Bran	42	**Fruits and Juices**	
Bran Chex	58	apple	38
Cheerios	74	apple juice	41
Corn Flakes	83	apricots	57
Cream of Wheat	70	banana	55
Crispix cereal	87	cantaloupe	65
Golden Grahams	71	cherries	22
Grape Nuts	67	cranberry juice	68
oatmeal	49	fruit cocktail	55
pancakes	67	grapefruit	25
PopTarts	70	grapefruit juice	48
puffed wheat	67	grapes	46
Raisin Bran	73	kiwi	53
Rice Krispies	82	mango	56
Shredded Wheat	69	orange	44

orange juice	52	peanuts	15
peach	42	popcorn	55
pear	37	potato chips	54
plum	39	pretzels	81
raisins	64	rice cakes	77
watermelon	72		

Legumes

baked beans	48
black beans	30
black-eyed peas	42
butter beans	30
chick peas	33
lentils, red	25
lima beans	32
pinto beans	45
red kidney beans	19

Pasta

capellini	45
fettucini	32
linguini	55
macaroni	45
spaghetti, white	41
spaghetti, wheat	37
tortellini	50

Rice/Grain

brown rice	55
couscous	65
instant rice	87
long grain rice	56
risotto	69

Snack Foods

corn chips	74
granola bars	61
NutriGrain bars	66

Soups

black bean	64
green pea	66
lentil	44
minestrone	39
split pea	60
tomato	38

Sports Bars/Drinks

Gatorade	78
Power Bar	58

Sugars and Spreads

glucose tablets	102
high fructose corn syrup (regular soda)	62
honey	58
strawberry jam	51
syrup	66
table sugar (sucrose)	64

Vegetables

French fries	75
potato, baked	85
potato, instant	83
potato, mashed	91
potato, boiled	88
carrots, boiled	49
carrots, raw	47
corn	46
sweet potato	44
tomato juice	38

Carbohydrate Replacement for Exercise

	Carbohydrate replacement (in grams) (per sixty minutes of physical activity)				
	50 lbs (23 kg)	100 lbs (45 kg)	150 lbs (68 kg)	200 lbs (91 kg)	250 lbs (114kg)
baseball	7–10	14–20	20–30	28–40	35–50
basketball	12–15	24–30	35–45	48–60	60–75
bowling	7–10	14–20	20–30	28–40	35–50
boxing (training)	18–22	37–43	55–65	74–86	92–107
carpentry	5–8	10–16	15–25	20–32	25–40
cycling (leisurely)	7–10	14–20	20–30	28–40	35–50
cycling (moderate)	12–15	24–30	35–45	48–60	60–75
cycling (racing)	25–28	50–56	75–85	100–112	125–140
dancing (ballroom)	5–8	10–16	15–25	20–32	25–40
dancing (lively)	8–12	17–23	25–35	34–46	42–57
farming (manual labor)	15–18	30–36	45–55	60–72	75–90
farming (w/ power eqpt)	2–5	4–10	5–15	8–20	10–25

	50 lbs (23 kg)	100 lbs (45 kg)	150 lbs (68 kg)	200 lbs (91 kg)	250 lbs (114kg)
field hockey	17–20	34–40	50–60	68–80	85–100
football	17–20	34–40	50–60	68–80	85–100
gardening	7–10	14–20	20–30	28–40	35–50
golf	7–10	14–20	20–30	28–40	35–50
grocery shopping	5–8	10–16	15–25	20–32	25–40
gymnastics	8–12	17–23	25–35	34–46	42–57
handball	15–18	30–36	45–55	60–72	75–90
hiking (w/ pack)	10–13	20–26	30–40	40–52	50–65
horse riding (gallop)	13–17	27–33	40–50	54–66	67–82
horse riding (trot)	10–13	20–26	30–40	40–52	50–65
horse riding (walk)	2–5	4–10	5–15	8–20	10–25
housework	3–7	7–13	10–20	14–26	17–32
jogging (3–5 mph)	12–15	24–30	35–45	48–60	60–75
judo/karate	23–27	47–53	70–80	94–106	117–132
machine tooling	5–8	10–16	15–25	20–32	25–40
mowing (push mower)	13–17	27–33	40–50	54–66	67–82
painting (walls)	7–10	14–20	20–30	28–40	35–50
racquetball	15–18	30–36	45–55	60–72	75–90
raking	5–8	10–16	15–25	20–32	25–40
rowing	13–17	27–33	40–50	54–66	67–82
running (12-min. miles)	13–17	27–33	40–50	54–66	67–82
running (10-min. miles)	20–23	40–46	60–70	80–92	100–115
running (8-min. miles)	28–32	57–63	85–95	104–116	125–140
running (6-min. miles)	38–42	77–83	115–125	154–166	192–207
skating (leisurely)	7–10	14–20	20–30	28–40	35–50
skating (intense)	18–22	37–43	55–65	74–86	92–107
skiing (cross-country)	18–22	37–43	55–65	74–86	92–107

	50 lbs (23 kg)	100 lbs (45 kg)	150 lbs (68 kg)	200 lbs (91 kg)	250 lbs (114kg)
skiing (downhill)	8–12	17–23	25–35	34–46	42–57
soccer	13–17	27–33	40–50	54–66	67–82
squash	18–22	37–43	55–65	74–86	92–107
swimming (slow)	12–15	24–30	35–45	48–60	60–75
swimming (fast)	22–25	44–50	65–75	88–100	110–125
tennis (doubles)	8–12	17–23	25–35	34–46	42–57
tennis (singles)	18–22	37–43	55–65	74–86	92–107
volleyball	8–12	17–23	25–35	34–46	42–57
walking (20-min. miles)	3–7	7–13	10–20	14–26	17–32
walking (14=min. miles)	8–12	17–23	25–35	34–46	42–57
weeding	5–8	10–16	15–25	20–32	25–40
weight training (circuit)	10–13	20–26	30–40	40–52	50–65

Index